HOMOEOPATHY IN PRACTICE

Homoeopathy
in
Practice

Dr Douglas Borland
MB, ChB, FFHom

Edited for publication by
Dr Kathleen Priestman
LRCP, MRCS, FFHom

BEACONSFIELD PUBLISHERS LTD
Beaconsfield, Bucks, England

First published in 1982

© Vida S. Borland 1982

British Library Cataloguing in Publication Data

Borland, Douglas M.
  Homoeopathy in practice.—(Beaconsfield
homoeopathic library; no. 5)
  1. Homoeopathy—Materia medica and therapeutics
  I. Title   II. Priestman, Kathleen G.
  615.5'32   RX601
  ISBN 0–906584–06–X

Set, printed and bound in Great Britain
in 10 on 12 point C.A.T. Times
by Billing and Sons Limited,
Guildford, London, Oxford, Worcester

Preface

I have found it very interesting to be able to help in preparing Dr Borland's manuscript for publication in book form. I attended a number of his original lectures myself, and possess the notes of other lectures attended by my former senior partner, Dr Agnes Moncrieff. I found these notes of great value during my years in general practice, and referred to them frequently, as well as to his books on *Children's Types* and *Pneumonias*.

The material in this book does not represent the entire balance of Dr Borland's hitherto unpublished lectures. It does, however, represent all of them that were taken down in shorthand. They are published here because Dr Borland's homoeopathic insight remains as important and as fresh today as it ever was. Wherever current practice has moved on from his time, notably in the availability of antibiotics and in the development of modern surgical techniques, I have edited the text to point this out.

One of the difficulties in homoeopathic prescribing is to distinguish between remedies with similar symptomatology, and Section II of this book examines a number of major groups of related remedies. The individual remedies are not presented in alphabetical order – Dr Borland frequently linked remedies by their common characteristics or differences, and excelled in leading on from one to another, as the reader will appreciate.

There are a number of occasions throughout the book where Dr Borland was explaining the use of homoeopathic remedies in a busy general practice surgery, and the word 'routine' is sometimes used. This is against the basic principle of homoeopathy, which is that an individual remedy is chosen for each patient according to the symptoms presented at the time. In practice there are certain common ailments which present with the same symptom picture in many individuals, so that the same remedy is indicated, and it is in this sense that the word 'routine' is used. Dr Borland warns the prescriber to be on the watch at all times for patients who do not fit the common symptomatology, and who therefore require another remedy.

Books on homoeopathic practice have sometimes been criticised for being too anecdotal, and for this reason most references to patients have been omitted. However, the picture of Lachesis, as demonstrated by Dr Borland's patient, is so typical that it has been included (Chapter 12).

This publication, small though it is, should be a most valuable tool in the hands of anyone using the homoeopathic method of treatment.

K. G. Priestman, LRCP, MRCS, FFHom

Explanation of Homoeopathic Terms

Potency

This is used to indicate the strength of the remedy. Samuel Hahnemann found in his original experiments on himself and on those testing the remedies – usually known as 'provers' – as well as when treating patients, that material doses of the substance he was using caused such unpleasant symptoms in the 'provers', and side effects in the patients, that he gradually reduced the dose. As he increased the dilution, he introduced a method of shaking the substance in dilution, finding by experience that the medicines used in this way had a more beneficial effect than when used in material doses.

The method of shaking he called succussion, and the result of dilution plus succussion he called 'potency'. In the past, the use of these very small doses has brought disbelief and ridicule to homoeopathy, but in these days of electron microscopy and the microchip, disbelief in the smallness of anything may well reflect more on the mind of the disbeliever than on the subject of his disbelief.

Hahnemann used two scales for his dilutions, the decimal and the centesimal. His method was as follows. Taking the original substance, he made a strong solution in either water or alcohol. The solution was then filtered and the filtrate was known as the 'mother tincture'. Using a new clean glass bottle and pipette for each step, one drop of the mother tincture was placed in the first bottle, and either 9 or 99 drops of alcohol (as pure as possible) were added. The bottle was corked and then shaken vigorously by striking it hard on a book or the palm of the hand ten times.

Then, taking one drop from this bottle, either 9 or 99 drops of the alcohol were added and the shaking or succussion repeated. This process was continued until the desired potency was reached.

The scale in which 9 drops of alcohol are used is denoted by the Roman numeral X and is known as the decimal scale. Where 99 drops of alcohol are used, the scale is designated by the Roman numeral C and known as the centesimal scale. That is, for example, Belladonna 1x, 2x, 3x, etc., or 1c, 2c, 3c, etc. The x potencies are known as 'low' potencies and also the lower scale of the c potencies. Potencies of the C scale have been taken to very high figures, even as far as the CM, and are known as high potencies from the 30c upwards. In modern times mechanical means are used for succussion. Hahnemann used his manual method as far as the 30c potency.

In this book, wherever no specific potency is mentioned, it is safe to use either 6c, 12c or 30c.

Modalities

These are the differences and modifications of symptoms. They are very important in relating the symptoms of the patient to the homoeopathic remedy, and concern the circumstances or conditions which make them better or worse. For example, a pain or sensation may be affected by:

1) Temperature, open air, weather, time of year, etc.;
2) Motion, touch, noise, position, eating, sleeping, etc.;
3) Time in 24 hours, etc.

Constitution, Constitutional Remedy or Type

Hahnemann was insistent that sickness in a person relates to the whole man and not to one particular part or organ of the body.

The people who tested or 'proved' remedies for him were asked to note every change or symptom that occurred in their thoughts, feelings and emotions, as well as physical sensations in every part of the body. These were carefully recorded under systematised headings, and gradually a pattern emerged for each remedy. This pattern became known as the 'drug picture' for that particular remedy.

It has been found that certain remedies are indicated very frequently, and that many people exhibit symptoms which correspond to the symptom picture or 'drug' picture of each of these remedies. Therefore they have become known as 'constitutional' remedies. The patients are said to have, for example, a Pulsatilla constitution or be a Pulsatilla type, or a Sulphur or Lycopodium type, according to which of these particular remedies their temperament most closely responds.

Unfortunately, over the years, it has become a common habit for homoeopathic doctors to speak of the remedies as if they were the patients and vice versa. It is to be understood, for instance, that the 'Kali Carb. backache with pain shooting down the thighs' may be used of a patient suffering from this condition, or also in a description of the Kali Carb. symptomatology.

To state that Pulsatilla is a certain person's constitutional remedy indicates that the individual's habitual personality resembles the 'picture' of Pulsatilla as it was brought out in the 'provers'. In any sickness where those Pulsatilla symptoms are intensified, Pulsatilla is the remedy that will bring the patient back into a state of health.

In acute conditions, patients may exhibit symptoms that indicate some remedy other than their constitutional one. In these cases, the prescription must always follow the homoeopathic law of similars. When the acute condition is resolved, it may well be that a dose of the patient's constitutional remedy will be needed to restore them to full health.

K. G. P.

Contents

Chapter 1

Injuries and Emergencies

SPRAINS AND DISLOCATIONS

Among the commonest minor surgical complaints seen in general practice are sprains, fractures and dislocations of all kinds. Much can be done to diminish the pain and shorten the period of disability. After an accident with general aching pain, whether it is a sprain, a dislocation or a fracture, where the part feels bruised with a dislike of movement which is painful, the first remedy to give is Arnica.

After a dislocation has been reduced but where there is still pain around the dislocated joint, or after a sprain where the patient is complaining of considerable pain, the affected joint being more comfortable when the patient moves it about but stiffening up when he keeps it still – i.e. so long as it is kept moving it is easier – give Rhus Tox.

In all acute cases, any potency may be used, 30c or higher. Give several doses, usually three doses two hours apart. That is the ordinary routine treatment.

One other allied condition is rupture of a muscle. This may occur with a severe sprain or dislocation. There are some indications for Arnica – very painful on movement, must keep as still as possible – and yet Arnica does not give relief. The patient finds it very difficult to move, and gets sharp pains in the torn muscle, rather than the bruised feeling of Arnica. A few doses of Bryonia help this condition just as much as Arnica helps the others. It is more commonly met with in back strain than anywhere else – a man has lifted something too heavy, something gives in his back and he is in great pain. A great many of these cases in general practice are a problem. Quite a few will respond to Arnica, but the majority respond very much better to Bryonia.

One warning: in a sprain with Rhus Tox. symptoms (where the affected area stiffens up with rest and is better for movement). In the typical warm-blooded, gentle Pulsatilla patient, Pulsatilla will be far more effective than Rhus Tox. Pulsatilla has exactly the same modalites as Rhus Tox., stiffens up in the same way, and Rhus Tox. does not seem to do much good. It is better to prescribe Pulsatilla in the first instance. Pulsatilla patients are rather the loose-jointed type and tend to get sprains. In spite of the Rhus Tox. symptoms, Rhus Tox. does not act in the typical warm-blooded gentle Pulsatilla type.

With persistent stiffness and weakness after sprains in the neighbourhood of a joint, Ruta can be given as a routine. Ruta has very much the Rhus Tox. modalities; the muscles tend to get stiff when not in use and to become easier with use. If Rhus Tox. has been given without effect, follow it up with Ruta, which will usually clear up the condition.

There are two remedies to consider for weakness of a joint following a sprain, or where there is a tendency to recurring dislocation. With a loose joint which tends to turn over and is weak, e.g. ankle, a few doses of Calcarea Carb. will strengthen the ligaments. Where the looseness and weakness of the joint is accompanied by a certain amount of stiffness as well as being easily dislocated, it will improve after a few doses of Strontium Carb. A patient who had received treatment for repeated subluxation of the right sacro-iliac joint without benefit was manipulated, and given Strontium Carb. Because the subluxation occurred when she used the brake on the car, she was also forbidden to drive for two months. She had no further trouble.

Muscular fatigue or general exhaustion from walking too far or driving too long can be helped by having a hot bath to which two tablespoonsful of Arnica tincture have been added, after which the individual feels completely refreshed.

For synovial effusion into a tendon sheath, or a pre-patella bursa or ganglion of the wrist, Ruta is almost specific. If a pre-patella bursa does not clear with Ruta it will usually do so on Apis.

FRACTURES

As an ordinary routine, start the patient on Arnica. There is considerable pain, effusion of blood and bruising, and the typical aggravation from movement. When dealing with a comminuted fracture, with a number of spicules of bone, particularly in the neighbourhood of a joint, or where a nerve has been injured by splinters of bone with pain shooting along the course of the nerve, Hypericum gives greater relief than Arnica. Where bony union is slow, callus formation can be stimulated by a few doses of Calc. Phos., the commonest remedy for slow union. The other possibility is Symphytum. These are often very helpful, as in many of these cases it is difficult to get any indication on which to prescribe, apart from the local injury.

HEAD OR SPINAL INJURY

For a head injury with concussion, or for a spinal injury, again with a degree of concussion, certain routine prescriptions can be given. In the case of head injury with mild concussion, the best prescription is Arnica. Where the concussion has been much more a spinal concussion rather than a head concussion, the best prescription is Hypericum. That is an immediate prescription. For concussion with persisting drowsiness with obviously increasing intra-cranial pressure, do not persist with Arnica but go on to Opium at once. When dealing with the later effects of concussion, the post-concussion headache, there are again certain routine prescriptions available. The most useful remedy is Natrum Sulph. Arnica is disappointing for a post-concussion headache. Natrum Sulph. is the commonest remedy for these cases, and the next most useful is Opium.

When dealing with the neuraesthenic symptoms which may be associated with a spinal concussion, the most commonly indicated remedy is Actea Racemosa, followed by Hypericum. (An alternative name for Actea Racemosa is Cimicifuga.) These remedies may all be given in the 30c potency.

SMALL WOUNDS AND LACERATIONS

For small wounds, lacerations and similar conditions there are three commonly indicated remedies. The commonest is Calendula. The ordinary homoeopathic routine of putting a Calendula dressing on wounds gives extremely good results, but they will be even better if Calendula in potency is given orally at the same time. Give three doses two hours apart of 30c or 200c potency. A wet Calendula dressing helps the bruising as well as the laceration.

With a wound involving any very sensitive area, such as the tips of fingers, beds of nails, or toes – where there is a great deal of pain, particularly shooting pains – before any red streaks indicate an infection, it can be prevented altogether by putting on a Hypericum dressing and giving Hypericum orally.

After a confinement, where there has been instrumental interference and damage to the coccyx, with coccygeal pain, or in a patient with a history of injury to the coccyx from a fall, Hypericum will relieve the pain. Hypericum is always indicated for the very sensitive areas plentifully supplied with nerves.

Lacerated fingers should be soaked in Hypericum lotion, followed by a Hypericum dressing, and Hypericum given in potency orally.

For a badly lacerated hand the same treatment should be given using Calendula. Not only does healing take place very rapidly but sepsis does not occur.

Arnica is most useful internally, but should not be used externally on any injury where the skin is broken as it may cause inflammation. Hamamelis will reduce bruising and is a safe external application in these conditions.

SEPSIS

For an inflamed area, very hot, puffy, tender, aggravated by hot applications which increase the swelling and congestion and increase the pain, with red streaks running up the lymphatics – as a routine, give Ledum. That is in the earlier stages. With a similar condition, but comfort from hot applications, the prescription is Hepar Sulph.

For a more virulent condition, with a rapid spread of sepsis and obvious early necrosis of tissue, there are three remedies to consider. Where there is very severe, stabbing pain accompanied by nervous excitement of the patient, the best prescription is Tarentula Cubensis. Where the infected area is dark purple, very hot, not so sensitive, throbbing rather than the stabbing pains of Tarentula Cub., the best prescription is Lachesis. In a typical Lachesis picture the whole part looks puffy and purple, purplish blue, swollen, with a tendency for the infection to spread very rapidly. Where there is a more advanced condition, with sloughing and great offensiveness, and oozing a quantity of black blood mixed up with pus, the best prescription is Crotalus Horridus.

For pustular eruptions after a septic infection the best prescription is Calc. Sulph.

The prescription for paronychia depends on the character of the pain, and on the response to heat and cold. The acute paronychia is acutely painful at the start and, during that extremely painful stage, if it is relieved by hot fomentations the best prescription is Hepar Sulph. If it is very much aggravated by hot applications, with swelling and tenderness, and stabbing, shooting pain, the best prescription is Apis. These two remedies in the majority of cases will abort an acute paronychia.

For a peri-anal inflammation, or inflammation round a faecal fistula, where there is any possibility of B. Coli contamination of an infection, give Rhus Tox. This seems to have an almost specific effect in these conditions.

(*Note*. Since the use of antibiotics, the very severe infections described by Dr Borland as needing Lachesis or Crotalus Horridus are rarely seen; also, if the *correct* homoeopathic remedy is given in the early stages of an infection the majority will clear up without the need for any more drastic measures. Ed.)

FAINTING

Where this is caused by the sight of blood, or by being in a crowded room, Ignatia is the remedy of choice. If the faintness is due to the heat and stuffiness of the room, and if standing is also intolerable – use Pulsatilla. Fainting due to shock will respond to Aconite.

INJURIES TO THE EYE – THE 'BLACK EYE'

If Arnica is given within a short time of the injury, there will be no 'black eye' – Arnica stops the effusion of blood. There may be some discolouration, but not the deep purplish swelling. If the patient is seen some time after the injury, with discolouration and swelling already present, there is a much better response from Ledum. With an injury to the eyeball itself Symphytum will relieve the pain more quickly and more definitely than Arnica.

EAR – ACUTE OTITIS MEDIA

In a case of acute otitis, with violent pain spreading to the mastoid region, there are three remedies to be considered. Aconite, Chamomilla and Capsicum.

Aconite

In a case where the symptoms have come on very suddenly, with a history of the patient having been out in a very cold north east wind, the patient is intensely restless, and the pains are very violent, usually burning in character. The patient is irritable, frightened, with a rising temperature and extreme sensitivity to touch. With that history, a few doses of Aconite will abort the acute inflammatory process.

Chamomilla

Another type of case is usually seen in children. There is not the same definite history of chill, although that may be present. The pain is even more intense and the patient is practically beside himself with pain, will not stay still, is as cross and as irritable as can be, with extreme tenderness, and gives the impression that nothing his parents do can satisfy him. After a few doses of Chamomilla the inflammatory process will rapidly subside.

Capsicum

In yet another type of case there is much more tenderness over the mastoid region, possibly a little swelling, with the ear beginning to look a little prominent on the affected side. The external ear is very red and there are very acute stabbing pains in the ear. Capsicum almost always clears up the condition which is a little relieved by hot applications, and where the patient is very sorry for himself, miserable, wanting to be comforted, probably a little tearful, but without the irritability of Chamomilla.

Pulsatilla, Mercurius, Hepar Sulph.

In addition to the above three remedies, bear in mind the possibility of a Pulsatilla child requiring a dose of Pulsatilla for the condition. And not infrequently one sees a case giving indications for Mercurius or Hepar Sulph.

ACUTE NEURALGIAS

For typical acute neuralgias, facial neuralgias or acute sciaticas, where relief is required as soon as possible, there are a number of remedies which may be used almost as a routine.

Consider acute facial neuralgia, acute trigeminal neuralgia; there are two outstanding drugs, Mag. Phos. and Colocynth. Spigelia is a third one which is sometimes indicated.

Magnesia Phosphorica
Take a case with very violent sharp stabbing pain, or twinges of pain running along the course of the nerve, coming on from any movement of the muscles of the face, very much aggravated by any draught of air, with extreme superficial tenderness over the affected nerve. If it is also much more comfortable from warmth – applied warmth – and much more comfortable from firm supporting pressure, such a case almost always responds to Mag. Phos. It does not really matter which branch of the nerve is involved, or which side, though it is more usually the right side than the left.

Incidentally, this does not apply to dental neuralgia. Dental cases are much more difficult and there are quite a number of remedies to choose from.

Colocynth
The same condition, with practically the same symptoms and the same modalities, affecting the *left* side, almost always responds to Colocynth.

The side usually determines the choice between Mag. Phos. and Colocynth, but occasionally either remedy may relieve neuralgias involving the opposite side.

Spigelia
In orbital neuralgia, with sharp stinging pains, or pain 'as if a red hot needle were stuck into it' – a very common description given by patients in these cases – the pains radiating out along the course of the nerve. In the majority of cases Spigelia will give relief.

One very useful point about Spigelia is that the patient sometimes says that, in spite of the burning character of the pain, there is a strange cold sensation in the affected area after it has been touched. This indicates Spigelia and no other remedy.

These three remedies are the most useful in a routine way for treating facial neuralgias.

As a rule, high potencies may be used. Sometimes, in these very painful conditions, a very high potency will aggravate the pain for 10 minutes or so, giving unnecessary suffering, so with acute pain a 30c potency is preferable.

POST-HERPETIC NEURALGIAS

Another group of conditions of the same type, the post-herpetic neuralgias, are sometimes very troublesome. In ordinary shingles neuralgia,
the patient comes in with acute burning pain along the course of an
intercostal nerve and gives a history that he has had a small crop of
herpetic blisters, very often so slight that he paid little or no attention to
it. Mag. Phos. will relieve if the same modalities are present as in the
facial neuralgias under Mag. Phos. But much more commonly these
post-herpetic cases respond to Ranunculus.

Ranunculus Bulbosus
The particular indications for this remedy are that the very sharp
shooting pains extend along the course of the intercostal nerve, that the
painful area is very sensitive to touch, and that the pain is induced or
aggravated by any movement, particularly by turning. If the condition
has been in existence for a little time, and the pains come on in wet
weather and are certainly aggravated by it, the patient becomes
extremely conscious of any weather change because it will start the
neuralgia again. That type of case responds in almost every instance to
Ranunculus.

Mezereum
There may be a few of these cases which have not responded to Ranunculus. There is much the same distribution of pain, much the same
modalities, but without the marked aggravation in wet weather. The
affected area is sensitive to any cold draught, particularly sensitive to
any bathing with cold water, and the pains are extremely troublesome
at night, with a marked hyperaesthesia over the affected area. These
cases will respond very well to Mezereum.

SCIATICA

Magnesia Phosphorica
There are helpful indications for certain remedies for another type of
neuralgia – the sciaticas. In a case of sciatica, pure sciatica, with no
indications except the ordinary classical symptoms of acute pain down
the sciatic nerve, which is aggravated by any movement, is very sensitive to cold and more comfortable if kept quiet and warm, then the
remedy indicated depends on which leg is involved. If it is a right-sided

sciatica, Mag. Phos. will relieve; if it is a left-sided sciatica use Colocynth. A large number of cases obtain almost immediate relief from either Mag. Phos. or Colocynth.

Kali Iodatum

In a few patients with sciatica, the pain increases the longer they keep still and they are compelled to move. There are two remedies which seem to relieve the majority of these cases. If the patient is a warm-blooded person, and if the sciatic pains tend to be more troublesome when warm – particularly warm in bed – and if better when moving about, Kali Iod. will give relief in the majority of instances.

Rhus Toxicodendron

If there are the same modalities with a patient who is sensitive to the cold, particularly if he is sensitive to damp as well as cold, and is more comfortable while moving about, Rhus Tox. will relieve a great many of the cases.

Gnaphalium

There are one or two curious indications which sometimes help in a sciatica with few other symptoms. For instance in a sciatica which has marked numbness associated with the acute sciatic pain, there are two remedies which cover most cases. One is Gnaphalium, which has this sensation of numbness associated with the pain and tenderness over the sciatic nerve, more markedly than any other remedy in the Materia Medica.

Plumbum

The second remedy which has this numbness associated with pain and tenderness of the sciatic nerve is Plumbum. The main indication for Plumbum is extreme constipation in addition to the pain and numbness.

ACUTE COLIC

Fortunately, the indications in acute colics are usually definite.

Aconite

A first attack of colic, whether it be biliary or renal, is a very devastating experience for the patient and he is usually terrified. The pains are extreme. If, in addition, the patient feels very cold and very anxious, feels faint whenever he sits up or stands up and yet cannot bear the room being hot, Aconite will very often give relief within a very short time.

Aconite is seldom indicated in repeated attacks. The patients begin to realise that although the condition is exceedingly painful it is not fatal, so the mental anxiety necessary for the administration of Aconite is not present, and without that mental anxiety Aconite does not seem to act.

Belladonna

Belladonna will bring almost immediate relief in a patient having repeated attacks of either biliary or renal colic, each one quite short in duration, developing suddenly, stopping suddenly, associated with a feeling of fullness in the epigastrium. The attacks are induced, or very much aggravated, by any fluids. The patient has a hot, red face, dilated pupils and a full bounding pulse.

Chelidonium

A patient who has had some liver symptoms for some time, just vague discomfort, slight fullness in the right hypochondrium, a good deal of flatulence, intolerance of fats, and who is losing weight, becoming sallow and perhaps slightly jaundiced, may be helped by Chelidonium. He develops an acute colic, an acute hepatic colic, with violent pain going right through to the back, particularly just at the angle of the right scapula. This pain subsides and leaves a constant ache in the hepatic region. Then the attack recurs, and again subsides. If the pains are relieved by very hot applications or drinking very hot water, Chelidonium will relieve these attacks very rapidly.

An X-ray of a patient with these symptoms will often show a number of gallstones. An X-ray taken again after an attack for which Chelidonium has been prescribed may show that the gallstones have passed, if they are small.

One or two other remedies are also very helpful for colic.

Berberis

Berberis often gives relief in colic, whether it is a renal colic or a gallstone colic. The outstanding point about the Berberis colics, of whatever type, is the fact that from one centre the pain radiates in all directions. In a renal colic – and when Berberis is indicated, it is more commonly a left-sided one than a right – the colicky pain may start in the renal region, or along the course of the ureter. There is one centre of acute pain and from that centre the pain radiates in all directions. In a hepatic colic the centre of acute intensity is the gallbladder, and from there the pain radiates in all directions, going through to the back, into the chest and into the abdomen.

In addition, with a renal colic there is an acute urging to urinate, and a good deal of pain on urination. A biliary colic is usually accompanied by a very marked aggravation from any movement. This is present to a slight extent in the renal colics, but less markedly. In both, the patient is very distressed and has a pale, earthy-looking complexion. The pallor is more marked in the renal cases, and there may be jaundice where there has been a previous gallstone colic.

No other remedy has the extent of radiation of the pain that is in Berberis.

With renal colic the urine usually contains a quantity of greyish white deposit which may be pus, and a quantity of amorphous material, usually phosphates, sometimes urates. It is not blood-stained. It is a very dirty-looking urine, but surprisingly inoffensive.

Magnesia Phosphorica

Two remedies frequently indicated for colics of any kind are Colocynth and Mag. Phos., whether the colic is uterine or intestinal, biliary or renal. The difficulty about these remedies is that they are almost identical. Always in their colics the pain is very extreme, and the patients are doubled up with it. In both cases the pains are relieved by external pressure, and in both cases the pains are relieved by heat. In Mag. Phos. there is rather more relief from rubbing than in Colocynth; Colocynth prefers steady, hard pressure. Their colics are intermittent. The patients get spasms of pain, which come to a climax and then subside.

There are one or two distinguishing points which help in making the choice. In Colocynth the patient is intensely irritable and impatient, wants immediate relief, and is liable to be violently angry if the relief is not forthcoming. In Mag. Phos. there is not the same degree of irritability, and the patient is distraught because of the intensity of the pain rather than being violently angry.

Another point that sometimes helps is that Colocynth tends to have a slightly coated tongue, particularly if it is the digestive tract that is upset, whereas Mag. Phos. usually has a clean tongue.

Both of these remedies have a marked aggravation from cold, a little more marked in Mag. Phos. than in Colocynth. For instance, Mag.

Phos. is exceedingly sensitive to a draught; Colocynth, though it likes hot applications, is not so extremely sensitive to cold air in its neighbourhood.

Another distinguishing point between the two is that in Colocynth there is a tendency to giddiness, particuarly on turning – especially on turning to the left – but this is not present in Mag. Phos.

Where there is a report that the colic – more commonly uterine than intestinal colic – has followed on an attack of anger, it is almost certainly Colocynth that will be required, and not Mag. Phos.

If the colic is the result of over-indulgence in cheese, Colocynth is indicated. If, on the other hand, the colic is the result of exposure to cold, either a dysmenorrhoea or an abdominal colic, it is much more likely to be Mag. Phos.

These are two of the most useful remedies in the Materia Medica for colics, and it is surprising how much relief can be obtained from their administration.

Dioscorea

This is another remedy which is very useful as a contrast to Mag. Phos. and Colocynth, and which has very much the same sort of pain – a very violent, spasmodic colic coming on suddenly, rising up to a head, then subsiding. It has the same relief from applied heat, and is sometimes more comfortable for firm pressure. But in contra-distinction to the other two remedies, instead of the patient's being doubled up with pain, they are hyper-extended; they will bend back as far as possible. Dioscorea is the only remedy which has that violent abdominal colic and gets relief from extreme extension.

Ipecacuanha

Ipecac. is one other remedy to consider for colic, and the indications for it are very clear and definite.

The character of the pain described in Ipecac. is much more cutting than the acute spasmodic pain occurring in most of the other colic drugs. But the outstanding feature is the feeling of intense nausea which develops with each spasm of pain, yet, in spite of the nausea, the patient has a clean tongue. Quite a number of adolescent girls have violent dysmenorrhoea. Characteristically they are rather warm-blooded people, and with the spasms of pain – they very often describe it as cutting pain in the lower abdomen – they become hot and perspiring, with acute nausea. They cannot stand up and any movement makes them worse. They have a perfectly clean tongue and a normal temperature. Very often Ipecac. will stop the attack as well as the tendency to dysmenorrhoea. It is one of the very useful remedies for colic, and tends to be overlooked.

Occasionally a case of renal colic, associated with the same intense nausea, will respond to Ipecac. but that is unusual. The indications for it are more commonly found in uterine cases.

Lycopodium, Opium and Raphanus

These are three remedies where the colic is accompanied by violent abdominal flatulence. It is always an intestinal colic in which they are indicated. It may be associated with a gallbladder disturbance – if so, it is much more likely to be Lycopodium than either of the other two. In all three there is a tendency for the flatulence to be held in various pockets in the intestines, giving irregular areas of distension. All three are likely to be indicated in post-operative abdominal distensions, or semi-paralytic conditions of the bowel. In a paralytic ileus following abdominal resection there are more likely to be indications for Raphanus and Opium than for Lycopodium; but if the paralytic condition is in the region of the caecum the indications are probably for Lycopodium rather than for the other two.

Lycopodium

That is the general distinguishing point. Then there are one or two extra points which help. For instance, in Lycopodium the colicky pain is likely to start on the right side of the abdomen, towards the right iliac fossa, and spread over to the left side, whereas in the other two it remains more or less localised in one definite area.

In Lycopodium there is liable to be a late afternoon period of extreme distress, the 4–8 p.m. period of aggravation of Lycopodium.

There is likely to be more rumbling and gurgling in the abdomen in Lycopodium, and more tendency to eructation, whereas in the other two the patient does not seem able to get the same relief. Where there is eructation the patients usually complain of a very sour taste in Lycopodium.

In Lycopodium, the patient is rather emaciated, with a sallow, pale complexion.

Opium

There are one or two points that lead to Opium instead of the other two. In Opium, there is apt to be a definite area of distension, and the patient will say that he gets a feeling as if everything simply churned up to one point and could not get past it. It is as if the intestinal contents were trying to squeeze past some obstructing band, or as if something were being forced through a very narrow opening.

Another point of selection is that with these attacks of colic the Opium patient tends to become very flushed, very hot, feels the bed distressingly hot and wants to push the blankets off. After the spasm has subsided he tends to become very pale and limp, and often stuporous.

The area of distension in Opium is likely to be in the centre of the abdomen rather than in the right iliac fossa, and it is one of the most commonly indicated drugs in a paralytic ileus.

Another point that sometimes indicates Opium is that when the pains are developing and coming up to a head the Opium patients become hypersensitive to noise.

Raphanus

The Raphanus type of post-operative colic is slightly different. Instead of getting the right side of the abdomen distended as in Lycopodium, or the swelling up in the middle as in Opium, in Raphanus there are pockets of wind. A small area comes up in one place, gets quite hard and then subsides, and a fresh small area does exactly the same. These pockets of wind may be in any part of the abdomen. In the acute attacks of pain the patients tend to get a little flushed, but not so hot as the Opium patients, and they do not have the tendency to eructation that is associated with Lycopodium. They do not seem to be able to get rid of their wind at all, either upwards or downwards. It is the small isolated pockets of wind coming up in irregular areas throughout the abdomen that give the indications for Raphanus.

Podophyllum

There are, of course, endless other remedies which have colic, but these are the ones that are most useful in emergencies. Podophyllum is one other which is useful to know, and it is mainly useful in biliary colics. It is also useful in intestinal colics associated with acute diarrhoea.

Where Podophyllum is indicated in biliary colic, there is always infection of the gallbladder. One of the first things indicating Podophyllum is that the temperature reaches a peak in the morning and not in the evening.

In addition, Podophyllum patients are always very miserable and depressed. They are disgusted with life. Podophyllum patients with biliary colic are always jaundiced.

In the majority of cases, the pain is not localised in the gallbladder area, but is more in the epigastrium, and tends to spread across from the middle of the epigastrium towards the liver region. The pains are described as twisting in character, and are very much aggravated by taking any food.

In Podophyllum, the subsidence of acute pain leaves a feeling of soreness in the liver region. Podophyllum patients lie stroking the liver area, which gives them a great sense of comfort.

Chapter 2

Headaches

Apis

Apis is indicated for headaches which occur as a result of emotional stress, excitement, or the checking of some discharge; for instance, catarrh checked suddenly by a potent spray, or a menstrual period checked by sudden shock or cold. The patients say that the headache starts in the morning as a violent, stabbing pain running through the head, associated with a general congestion throughout the whole head. They are flushed, with facial congestion and usually slight swelling. There is often some conjunctival congestion, the eyes are unduly bright and the pupils are dilated. They are excited and have an intense aggravation from heat. They get violent shooting pains through the head, from side to side, and aggravated by movement. These headaches are usually relieved by pressure and cold applications, yet the whole scalp becomes tender to touch due to the severe pain. The skin, particularly of the forehead, is moist. In addition, these patients have the usual Apis general nervous excitement, irritability and dislike of being disturbed or interfered with.

Belladonna

At first sight the headaches are very similar to the Apis headaches. They come on under the same circumstances, but there are other conditions which also cause them. For instance, any heat, particularly of the sun; and under the opposite conditions, exposure to cold. Sensitive people may get a headache from washing the hair and not drying it properly before going out, or after a haircut. The headaches are also caused by emotional shock or fright.

The appearance is not unlike that of Apis. The patients have a hot head and are very flushed, but it is a much brighter flush than in Apis, and there is not the same degree of puffiness of the face as in Apis, or the same degree of conjunctival congestion. There is intense photophobia and, with the headaches, they are incredibly sensitive to any motion, jar or mis-step. With the pain there is a general pulsation; it may be temporal or it may be all over the head. On stooping, it is as if the whole head were throbbing. Another thing that distinguishes Belladonna from Apis, although there is such intense heat of the head, is that the patients themselves are chilly and like to be covered up warmly. They do not have the Apis desire for cold applications on the head, and the head is not damp but very definitely dry. In spite of the aggravation from motion, they do not want to lie down. They like to be propped up, often with their heads well back, because there is a degree of tension in the posterior cervical mucles, and bending the head back gives relief.

The headache comes on at 4 or 5 o'clock in the afternoon and persists right through the night. The patients are much worse from using the eyes, particularly from turning the eyes or attempting to follow any movement. Very often they not only complain of pulsation in the head but the pulse is visible beating in the temple. The headache is relieved by firm pressure. There may be a marked degree of mental excitement – it is always present in children, and children suffering from exposure to the sun are almost certain to become delirious during the night.

Bryonia
Bryonia gives a different picture altogether. The headaches usually come on during the night, patients waken with a headache, but are not acutely conscious of it until they get up and begin moving about. They complain of a dull aching pain in the frontal region, as if deep in the front part of the brain, and this aching, heavy pain tends to spread right through the head into the occiput. The pain comes on when getting up in the morning, and persists throughout the whole day. A Bryonia headache may develop during the day, but as the result of some definite exciting cause. The commonest time is during the night. Generally, the patient has been rather over-doing it the day before, and has been up late, possibly drinking too much or eating too much – more likely over-eating than drinking – and in the morning has a typical Bryonia headache. Sometimes a typical Sepia comes up to town for a day's shopping, enjoys a visit to a theatre, and then will often develop a Bryonia headache before the day is out. Another thing which will cause a Sepia patient to develop a Bryonia headache is ironing; she gets hot, tired and headachey, and if given Bryonia the headache will be relieved very rapidly.

With the aching pain in the head there is a feeling of heaviness and heat, accompanied by a general feeling of chilliness and particularly cold hands and feet. This is unlike ordinary Bryonia patients, who are generally worse from heat.

During the headaches the eyes are heavy, and any use of them is very painful. If the headache is really severe, the head is very tender. Even the hair is sensitive to touch, but in spite of this the headache is relieved by firm pressure.

Like all the other Bryonia symptoms the headaches are very much worse from motion, or jarring. The patients are irritable and, with a headache, cannot bear talking to people; the effort of speaking makes the headache so much worse. If the headache is associated with any dietetic indiscretion, the bowels frequently fail to act on the morning of the headache. In other words, the old custom of taking an aperient after an unwise and excessive dinner was not at all a bad idea. On stooping, the patients experience a sensation as if the whole head would burst. Lying still and putting cold applications on the forehead will give relief.

China Sulphuricum

A China Sulph. headache is always associated with a digestive upset. The typical patients are the rather delicate, chronic dyspeptics. Sometimes people of this type who have had a rather strenuous week or two, and become exhausted, will develop a violent headache. It starts in the back of the neck, spreads over the head and settles in the forehead, and they complain of a violent aching pain. One definite diagnostic point is the appearance of the patients, who give the impression that they are just about to vomit. They are pale, clammy, sweaty, look unwell, and have the peculiar greyish-green colour that people get prior to vomiting. Associated with the headaches, such patients get intense, troublesome flatulence, and are constantly bringing up small amounts of slightly sour-tasting gas. They develop an artificial hunger, feeling hungry all the time, but food does not relieve them. Lycopodium patients have the same sensation, but their headache is relieved by food and the flatulence is relieved by eructation, while in China Sulph. patients it is not so. China Sulph. patients get marked relief from pressing the head against something cold, although in general they are definitely chilly. They want to keep the head as still as possible, because the pain is very much aggravated by turning the head or using the eyes; it is also very much aggravated by moving about in the open air.

Cocculus

There are two circumstances in which indications for Cocculus are present. First, the patients develop a very typical headache after a long journey. Second, the headache is one which starts after a period of strain. For instance, a mother who has been looking after a sick child and has had no sleep for a couple of nights, or a businessman who has been through a crisis, or round about examination time in people who are studying hard and getting too little sleep.

Cocculus people will often say that they feel dead tired, exhausted, and rather giddy. They have a peculiar sensation of the head being empty and numb, followed immediately by a sensation as if it would burst with pain, as if the skull were opening and shutting. The pain is very severe, particularly at the back of the head, and the intense pain is almost always accompanied by nausea and may go on to actual vomiting. It is aggravated by sleep; after having a little sleep they always waken with the headache much worse. It is greatly aggravated by any stimulant such as coffee, alcohol and especially tobacco. During the headaches they develop intolerance for hot rooms, and want cold air. When the pain is severe in the occiput, the back of the head becomes extremely tender and they cannot bear to lie down. If the headache has continued for some time, particularly the occipital type, it extends down the back of the neck and the patient feels as if a tight cord were pulling the head back and down the spine. The pain is aggravated by motion, particularly any sudden motion, also by mental effort, and by any use of the eyes.

Gelsemium

It is a little difficult to know whether to place Gelsemium among the acute or the chronic remedies, as it has acute headaches but also recurring periodical headaches.

In the acute type, the headache comes on in association with some other disturbance, such as an acute cold, or after exposure to cold, with signs of acute coryza. There is always some degree of disturbance of sight; it may be simply a slight haziness of vision, it may be diplopia, it may be partial blindness, or it may be a flickering before the eyes.

With the headaches the patients have a very heavy, sleepy, drowsy appearance, and they always have some degree of heaviness of the eyelids, with difficulty in keeping the eyes open. They say they feel heavy and sleepy with the pain. Usually the headaches start during the forenoon and subside towards evening. If the patients lie down, as a rule the headache becomes worse at first, but if they continue lying it gradually subsides. The pain is usually a boring pain, often situated in the frontal region, most often over the right eye, and associated with a

sensation of coldness at the back of the head. When the headache is
very severe it produces a sensation of faintness. If the patients can get a
good sleep this normally clears the headache; or, at least, it eases the
pain. It is made much worse by motion and there is always some degree
of photophobia. As the pain begins to ease there is an increase in the
amount of urine excreted – this is a strong indication for prescribing
Gelsemium. Vomiting will also practically always relieve the headache.

Glonoinum

Glonoinum, the next of these remedies, has a very definite symptom
picture, the typical picture of sunstroke or heat stroke.

The first impression is that it is very like Belladonna but much more
severe. There is a very marked degree of congestion, but the patient has
a rather duskier colour. Belladonna patients are bright red, whereas
Glonoinum patients are purple. There is rather more puffiness of the
face in Glonoinum than in Belladonna. The skin is moist in Glonoinum
and there is not the dry heat of Belladonna.

The complaint of the patient is always that the head feels as if it is
going to burst, the whole head feels full, and the skull feels as if it were
actually swelling. Accompanying the headaches there is usually some
degree of eye disturbance. There are flashes of light before the eyes, or
everything seen is red, or there may be temporary loss of sight. The
pains in the head are very much aggravated by any motion or jarring
or by any physical exertion. These all make the head throb and feel as if
it would burst. There is amelioration from ice-cold applications and
from keeping quite still. In typical cases of sunstroke, the patients sit
with their elbows on their knees and the head gripped in their hands.
They will answer if spoken to but will not look up, as they keep their
head as still as possible.

Occasionally, after exposure to the sun, a headache of that type
occurs as a hemicrania instead of the usual generalised headache.
There may then be a peculiar symptom – a flushing of one side of the
face with dilatation of the vessels on that side, and comparatively little
on the other side. Sometimes these patients give a history of having had
sunstroke in the tropics, and they are now liable to get the same type of
headache in summer in more temperate climates, though not so
severely. The headaches start at sunrise, are worst at mid-day, and tend
to go with sunset. As a rule, Glonoinum will altogether cure the
headache in a patient with this history of sunstroke and this time
modality.

Melilotus

Occasionally a patient gives all the symptoms of Glonoinum, but does not respond to it at all. Melilotus has almost the same symptoms as Glonoinum, except that there is a little more excitement in Glonoinum, and a little more dullness, sleepiness and duskiness in Melilotus. They are rather more sensitive to thundery weather than Glonoinum, which has no definite thunder aggravation at all. Another point is that Melilotus and Glonoinum patients describe their discomfort slightly differently. In Glonoinum the whole head feels as if it is going to burst, it is so full. In Melilotus it feels as if a vessel would burst inside the head. So, if headache of this type does not respond to Glonoinum, give Melilotus. The most useful potency for the patient to carry with him is 30c – otherwise the 200c may be given.

Iris

It is not easy to decide whether to include Iris with the acute remedies or not. The headaches are as acute as any, but they also tend to be recurrent. The patients give a history of getting over-tired, and they tend to get a day or two when they are particularly tired, heavy and sleepy before the headache. Then they wake up at 2 or 3 a.m. and know that the headache is coming on. It is always preceded by disturbance of vision, hemianopia, fortification spectra or something similar. The attack usually develops – and this is a differentiating point from a number of other remedies – with the eye disturbances, vomiting and nausea, before the headache actually begins. The type of vomit is very suggestive. It is similar to Kali Bich. – white, tenacious, stringy fluid, often quite tasteless. After some hours the patient develops a violent headache, with a feeling of heat and fullness in the head, and an absolutely stupefying, stunning sort of pain. This pain is usually worse on the right side, but so severe that it involves practically the whole head. It is worse on keeping still, and better by moving about gently. It is slightly relieved by a draught of cool air, though it is aggravated by cold air; cool air is definitely comforting. The patient is liable to get a peculiar boring pain just in the middle of the epigastrium if the vomiting has gone on for more than two or three hours. It is in the pancreatic region, and it is interesting that Iris patients are sensitive to sugar. If they are over-tired they tend to get a sugar hunger. Then they are apt to indulge in too many sweets, and the result is that they develop a typical Iris headache. This is quite a usual history, and is easy to link up with the pancreatic pain.

Another point about the Iris headache is that each attack develops at exactly the same hour of the twenty-four hours.

The indications for Iris are always found in a very definite type of patient. They are artistic, thin, delicate and nervous,and they are usually very charming people to meet.

Lachesis

Lachesis headaches occur most frequently during the menopause. In addition they occur from exposure to heat, sun, fright, shock or grief.

Patients usually complain of a sensation of a rush of blood to the head. This is followed by a pressing, burning pain, most commonly in the vertex, with a sensation of a weight on the head, or a feeling that the head is expanding because it is too full. Another sensation is an acute pulsation, particularly in the temples. Associated with their headaches they get a flushed face, even a dusky appearance, accompanied by emotional excitement.

With these headaches patients are very sensitive to motion, any movement increases the feeling of fullness, and the pain is aggravated by pressure. The patient likes to sit propped up, as any stooping or lying down increases the congestion and increases the pain. Also, emotional excitement of any kind increases the congestion and the headache, and brings on the pain. Any stimulant may precipitate a bad headache, and Lachesis patients are peculiarly sensitive to them when a headache threatens.

The headache is aggravated by sleep. This is increased during the menopause, when a slight headache will become a blinding one after sleep. This is greater the longer the sleep – after a doze it is not quite so severe.

These patients often develop flooding during the menopause, and the flow always ameliorates the headache very quickly. Occasionally with the violent headaches and congestion they get shortness of breath, and the usual Lachesis sense of constriction, but this is by no means constant.

Magnesia Phosphorica and Silica

Mag. Phos. has two definite types of headache. One is a superficial, neuralgic headache, with neuralgic pains shooting over the head along the course of the superficial nerves of the head. The other is a very severe deep-seated headache starting at the back of the head, spreading through it and settling over the right eye. This Mag. Phos. headache can be confused with Silica, in which the pain also tends to develop in the back of the neck, spreads right over the head, and settles over the right eye, and in which there is also marked aggravation from cold. In Silica, however, there is no relief from pressure – in fact, wearing a tight hat is often enough to bring on a Silica headache. The types of patient will also probably be different. Silica patients tend to be fine skinned, fine haired and small boned. Mag. Phos. patients tend to have a fairly well developed bony framework, they are rather emaciated and somewhat sallow and greyish complexioned, and have dark rings under the eyes.

The two types of Mag. Phos. headaches come on under different circumstances. The acute neuralgic ones come on from cold and exposure to cold winds, though sometimes also after extreme nervous strain with the history of exposure to cold. The deep-seated headache always occurs in exhausted patients in poor health, and these tend to be recurring. These recurring headaches tend to be worse from 9 to 11 o'clock in the morning and from 4 to 8 o'clock in the evening. With the neuralgic type the patients are usually pale, but with the chronic type of headache the patients tend to be rather flushed. They develop marked sensitiveness to touch, whether it is a neuralgic or a deep-seated headache, and, although they develop this superficial hyper-aesthesia, the headache is definitely relieved by firm pressure. They are extremely sensitive to cold, no matter which type of headache they have. They are also better from warm applications, so much so that they have a dread of uncovering the head for fear of any cold air blowing on it.

Students are particularly liable to develop Mag. Phos. headaches. There are two types of students' headaches, the commonest being the one that tends to develop over the forehead just above the eyes, associated with intense eye weariness. The other develops in the back of the head and spreads right through it to settle over the right eye. This is the one that is so difficult to distinguish from Silica.

Nux Vomica

The Nux Vomica headache is the typical 'morning after' headache due to alcoholic excess, although it occurs from over-eating as well as over-drinking. The patients complain of a general fullness in the head with a feeling of congestion and pressure. The pressure is usually on the upper part of the head, often in the higher frontal region. The headache is always associated with constipation, but is not necessarily accompanied by vomiting. One useful point, which distinguishes it from the Bryonia headache, is that the Nux Vomica headache is present on waking in the morning, whereas the Bryonia headache does not come on until the patients begin moving about.

Nux Vomica patients are usually very chilly during their headaches and always bad tempered. They do not like to be spoken to or disturbed, and they hate to move. If they have to go and work, the headache is very much aggravated by any mental concentration. They usually have a feeling of nausea and if they force themselves to take food it aggravates their headache. This is a useful distinguishing point from Lycopodium, when the headache is eased by taking a little food. If Nux Vomica patients have to go out in the morning into the cold air they immediately get an increase of the frontal headache. Any noise greatly aggravates the headache and they are very irritable. The headaches are better from lying down, and aggravated by taking any stimulant, such as wine or coffee.

One clinical point – most of these patients tend to be thin and dark. With the same history in a fair patient and little response to Nux Vomica, consider Lobelia. Nux Vomica is much more likely to be useful in thin, irritable, dyspeptic, dark patients.

Sanguinaria and Gelsemium
The remedy most likely to be confused with Sanguinaria is Gelsemium. The actual pain in Sanguinaria is rather more intense than in Gelsemium. Instead of the general dusky, heavy, sleepy appearance of Gelsemium, there is more likely to be a generalised flush of the cheeks in Sanguinaria. Again, in Gelsemium the patients usually feel chilly down their backs, whereas in Sanguinaria they are likely to get a distressing, uncomfortable, burning heat of the palms of the hands and soles of the feet.

The patients complain that the whole head feels as if it were full of blood and as if it would burst, or they have a feeling of fullness at the back of the eyes, as if they were being pushed forward. This is similar to the symptoms in Bryonia, but in Bryonia the sensation is rather different. It is a sensation of fullness in the forehead with a feeling of weight settling right down on top of the eyes, making the lids feel heavy. As a rule, the pain of a Sanguinaria headache starts in the occipital region and spreads over the whole head. It tends to be rather more intense on the right side. With violent headaches there is not infrequently tenderness of the face and neuralgic pain involving the whole of the upper jaw. The headaches come on in the morning and last until evening, and a good night's sleep generally clears them. The patients are more comfortable keeping as quiet as possible in a dark room. Another distinguishing point between Sanguinaria and Gelsemium is that there is no definite urinary increase at the end of the headache in Sanguinaria, whereas in Gelsemium the patient knows that the pain is about to subside because the urinary output is increased.

There often tends to be a certain amount of periodicity in these headaches, usually about a seven-day recurrence.

Spigelia

Spigelia is only called for in cases of typical nervous headaches. They usually start at the back of the head, spread up over it, and settle over the left eye or in the left temple. The pain is pulsating, throbbing, and stabbing. Associated with the headaches, the patients get some degree of pain in the eyes, often more marked in the left. It is described as a sensation as if the eye was too big for its socket. This is a distinguishing point from Sanguinaria, in which there is a feeling of the eye being pushed out. The patients complain of stabs of pain radiating back through the head, coming on in the morning, usually about mid-day, and tending to decrease towards evening. The pain is aggravated by using the eyes for any purpose at all, as well as by motion in general, particularly jarring, sudden motion. The head is sensitive to touch and the pain is increased by noise. The most comfortable position is lying on the right side – not the painful side – and keeping the head and shoulders supported with pillows. These headaches usually come on after some emotional upset.

Theridion

Theridion headaches usually start about puberty, though they also occur round about the menopause. There are one or two outstanding features about them. The pain is a pressing one just at the back of the eyes, and from there it spreads backwards through the head. Associated with it the patients have a definite and intense giddiness which is particularly marked when they close the eyes, whatever their position. The giddiness is accompanied by nausea. With frontal headaches, patients usually want to keep their eyes closed – with Theridion patients it is exactly the opposite.

These patients are abnormally sensitive to noise, which causes throbbing pain in the head, shooting to the face and down the spine. With most of their headaches they develop hyper-sensitivity all down the spine to touch and jarring. The headaches are relieved by lying down and keeping quiet. This is the patients' most comfortable position.

When considering Theridion, the main points are giddiness, nausea, pain on closing the eyes, hyper-sensitivity to noise, and the headache occurring either at the start or cessation of menstruation.

Two other remedies should be considered. They are very difficult to distinguish and they come on in the same type of people and under the same circumstances – Aconite and Ignatia.

Aconite

With either of these remedies the patients are liable to headaches as a result of definite emotional crisis, or fear, or excitement. These are the commonest causes, but in Aconite, in addition, headaches may occur from exposure to either heat or cold. There the similarity ends.

During their headaches, Aconite patients always suffer from extremely violent pain, so severe that it makes them almost delirious. A typical instance of this is an Aconite sunstroke, with sudden onset of very violent, agonising pain, intense fear, and marked excitement. The patients complain of burning, throbbing, tearing pains in the head and a feeling of congestion as if the brain was too big for the skull and would burst out through the front of the head. They get marked congestion of the whole head and face. The headache is aggravated by light, noise, heat or any motion. During their headaches they get the usual Aconite restlessness, fear and anxiety, and yet any movement will increase the pain in their head. The indications for Aconite are the history of exposure, acute emotional crisis and fright, also the intense emotional excitement of the patient and the intense fear; it is a most violent condition.

Ignatia

In Ignatia, on the other hand, the indications are the general Ignatia make-up of the patient, with the history of emotional crisis as the result of disappointment or grief, though occasionally the cause of the headache will be a fright. They do not suffer from headaches which are due to exposure, and they are not liable to sun headaches, though a headache may develop during the course of a cold.

The pain is nothing like so violent as in Aconite. Ignatia patients are always the sensitive, slightly hysterical type. Anyone of that type who has suffered a severe disappointment and spent the day weeping is almost certain to need Ignatia to relieve a headache before night. With their headaches they often have an artificial hunger, a feeling of emptiness in the stomach. For a time their headaches are rather better from taking food; but it is only for a very short time and quite soon after eating the headache returns with increased severity.

Usually the headaches are most troublesome in the forehead, and patients complain of a general fullness and congestion in the forehead.

If they are disturbed at all, or have to move or talk, they get spasmodic pains over a small area of the head. In that condition they get relief from lying on the painful side. They develop a certain amount of nausea, and during the headache they become sensitive to coffee, tobacco or alcohol. They are better from keeping absolutely quiet. The headache is ameliorated by pressure, and the patients are very sensitive to noise or light, and particularly to looking up. Any increase of emotional disturbance will greatly aggravate the headache, also any excitement or talking, and particularly contradiction.

The different types of headaches tend to recur more at one season of the year than another. For instance, Bryonia headaches are much more frequently met with in winter. Of course, during a period of financial crisis or at examination times, the nerve strain headaches are common. After dietary indiscretions Nux Vomica will probably be indicated.

Chapter 3

Sore Throats

Rhus Toxicodendron and Arnica

In a patient with an uncomfortable sore throat after tonsillectomy, with stiffness of the muscles of the throat in the morning, Rhus Tox. is the remedy to prescribe. If after the operation there is complete inability to swallow, also pain of head and neck, Arnica is indicated; it eases the pain and the inflammation decreases. If the patient has stiffness and swelling in the throat on waking, and a quantity of sticky mucus in the throat, with pain on first swallowing, becoming easier if persisted in, again Rhus Tox. is indicated. With these two remedies, Arnica and Rhus Tox., the patient will improve very quickly. Rhus Tox. is not indicated the first day – it is usually Arnica. On the second day Rhus Tox. may be needed. There is a tendency to prescribe routinely – then the odd case occurs and the usual remedies are no use at all. One case in ten requires a different remedy, and the majority of the tenth cases need one of the Mercurius salts. These patients have a very inflamed throat with exudate on the surface and a pale tongue. They feel alternately hot and cold and are sweating slightly, with a raised temperature. They are much worse from any hot fluid, and cold drinks ease them. The breath is offensive. The condition should improve rapidly if Merc. Sol. is prescribed.

If there is slight bleeding from the throat, it is better to give Merc. Cyanide rather than Merc. Sol. These remedies will deal with almost all post-tonsillectomy cases.

(*Note*. Mercurius Solubilis and Mercurius Vivus are interchangeable, and are abbreviated as Merc. Ed.)

Aurum Muriaticum

This may be required in patients with a history of a cold and persistent sore throat. There is congestion, enlargement of the tonsils, redness of the fauces, and possibly ulcers in the mouth or throat, or a history of ulceration during the acute stage of the cold. There is a quantity of sticky mucus in the throat, which is very difficult for the patients to clear away. They cannot get the throat quite free, and the effort to clear it is painful. There is a sensation of heat round the tonsils and in the upper part of the pharynx, and the throat is much more comfortable after taking food. There may be enlargement of the glands in the neck. The patients are rather flabby and pale, and the tongue is swollen. They are chilly and have rheumatic pains, mainly a feeling of stiffness, particularly at the back of the knees, as if the hamstrings were a bit short, or they have stiffness in the muscles of the shoulders, elbows and particularly the hands. There is a tendency to sweat on their extremities, particularly their feet. Three or four doses of Aurum Mur. should clear the symptoms.

Baryta Muriaticum

The patients give a history of frequent colds which always affect the throat. On examination the patient is flushed, the lips are rather dry and there is a slightly coated tongue, white and rather greasy, and a heavy breath rather than an offensive one. The throat is congested, and the tonsils are enlarged and somewhat dusky in colour. As a rule there is a tendency for the right side to be more involved than the left. Associated with this enlargement of the tonsils and the fact that there is a recurring sore throat, there is a tendency to obvious enlargement of the veins of the posterior pharyngeal wall. It is covered with a good deal of mucus and secretion. The patients complain of difficulty in swallowing, as if there was a plum in the throat. Usually it is not very painful, but sometimes there is pain shooting up into the ear. That pain is relieved by a sip of cold water. There is enlargement of glands under the angle of the jaw. The patients usually say that the symptoms start in the evenings and that they have had a very uncomfortable night – they were hot and damp during the night and had very little sleep. They are often more comfortable in the morning and often have quite a good appetite in spite of the sore throat. These patients will respond to Baryta Mur. They may run a temperature up to 38 5°C.

Calcarea Sulphurica

In the very rare event of a quinsy, the drug most commonly indicated after it has been incised is Calc. Sulph. Instead of the white-coated tongue, the tongue tends to become yellow at its base. The patient's temperature is higher than when Baryta Mur. is indicated. He perspires more freely and is more flushed in appearance, possibly a little more dusky. The throat is obviously more swollen, more oedematous and darker red than the typical Baryta Mur., and the choking sensation is definitely worse – it is a real choking instead of just the plum sensation of Baryta Mur. The glands of the neck become more enlarged and the patients tend to be acutely thirsty. Calc. Sulph. patients want air, and are uncomfortably hot, whereas Baryta Mur. are hot in the night, but not uncomfortably hot. The extremities are hot, more especially the feet, and patients often complain of itching of the hands and feet.

Dulcamara

This is another remedy which may be difficult to identify, but which is quite frequently indicated. The typical history is of the patient having been chilled and within a short time developing an uncomfortable, painful throat, associated with a good deal of hoarseness. On examination, the throat is red, dark red in colour, rather shiny and dry, with profuse post-natal catarrh. The patients complain of a yellow, slimy discharge, particularly in the mornings. The tongue is dry and rough and the patients develop herpetic spots about the lips. There is a tendency for patches of urticaria to occur, with itching aggravated from heat and better from cold, and worse from scratching. Unlike the ordinary tingling of urticaria, it begins to burn if it has been scratched. There are general aching pains and general heat of the head and body, with coldness of the extremities. With these symptoms the patients should respond to Dulcamara.

Guiacum

This is very useful in acute attacks of tonsillitis which have developed suddenly, with painful glands of the neck. The pain in the neck and in the tonsils is very much more comfortable from external pressure, and the patients will sit up in bed holding the neck. The temperature is always high. The tongue is always furred. As a rule the patients are obviously toxic – the face is puffy and the colour ashen. They tend to have dilated pupils, which is suggestive of this remedy. They all have joint pains and they may get a little swelling, particularly about the fingers, and are more uncomfortable when hot, so they keep their hands outside the bedclothes. Rather than acute pain in the throat they complain of intense heat. They complain of headache, with a very severe, intense pain at the nape of the neck. There is a night aggravation from about 6 o'clock in the evening till about 4 o'clock in the morning. These symptoms will clear with Guiacum.

Aethusa

This remedy is required for the more chronic sore throat, the chronic pharyngitis. The patients complain of a hot uncomfortable throat, of which they are very conscious all the time. The condition never quite clears, and every now and then the symptoms become worse, and when troublesome there is always increased catarrh, particularly post-nasal. It occurs most commonly in patients who have had their tonsils removed in childhood, so they have no definite tonsillitis. On examination of the throat there is an atrophic condition of the mucous membrane, which is covered with streaks of white or yellowish mucus, and possibly the pharyngeal wall is mapped by dilated, often tortuous veins. The patients will remark that on attempting to clear this rather adherent mucus they very often get a little bleeding from the back of the throat. They are sensitive to cold, damp air, which makes the throat much worse, and may also have a nondescript flatulent dyspepsia. They may have quite a high colour, with a tendency to rather dilated veins on the cheeks and a tendency to swelling of the extremities. In this condition the remedy most likely to help is Aethusa.

Mercurius

In Mercurius cases there is a more septic type of throat than in simple tonsillitis. The patient's mouth tends to be dirty, the tongue heavily coated with the impression of being swollen, and it may show the imprints of the teeth on the sides. The outstanding indication is its offensiveness.

Mercurius throats are extremely painful. The patients often complain of the throat feeling very dry in spite of the fact that there is always very marked salivation. Patients will often say that the saliva trickles out of the mouth at night when they are asleep, although the throat feels hot and dry.

They complain of the throat feeling very full. It is accompanied by stiffness in the neck, and the tonsillar and cervical glands are enlarged. Any effort to swallow is extremely painful. On examination, the throat is swollen and dusky red, with a quantity of dirty mucus stretching over the tonsils.

At a slightly later stage, small patches of darker red appear over the generally congested tonsils. These Mercurius throats may go on to an acute quinsy, with isolated dusky spots tending to coalesce, forming a bulging area – a typical quinsy throat.

Mercurius patients always perspire. They feel hot, and yet when uncovered they promptly become chilly and cover up again. There may be small superficial ulcerated patches on the tonsil or there may be deeper pus formation.

That is the typical Mercurius picture.

Mercurius Cyanatus
In Merc. Cy. the throat is a little more dirty, with a greater tendency to ulceration. There is less tendency to abscess formation, and if swabbed, a Merc. Cy. throat will almost certainly bleed.

Another distinguishing point in the Cyanide is that an area of ulceration will frequently have a very bright red area of demarcation, as if it has been edged round with a red ink pen.

But so far as the choice between Merc. and Merc. Cy. is concerned, it is purely a question of intensity – the Cyanide is more virulent, more rapid in its onset, more ulcerative in type, and there is much more tendency to bleed.

Mercurius Iodatus Rubrum or Mercurius Iodatus Flavus
Occasionally a patient with indications for Merc. does not respond sufficiently well. The condition responds up to a point, but not really satisfactorily, so one of the other Mercurius salts, either Merc. I. R. or Merc. I. F. should be considered.

If a case is not responding very well, with definite Mercurius indications and affecting the right side, better results may be obtained from Merc. I. F. than from Mercurius. If, on the other hand, it mainly involves the left side of the throat, it may be found that Merc. I. R. sometimes takes up the work in place of Mercurius, just as Merc. I. F. does for the right side. It is a help to remember that the Rubrum, the R, applies to the left not to the right.

Phytolacca
The next most useful remedy for these throats is Phytolacca.

Phytolacca patients have a very similar type of throat to that of Mercurius, but there are one or two points which distinguish it. In Phytolacca there is a tendency for the glandular enlargement to be a little more obvious than it is in Mercurius, and not infrequently it will extend to the cheek, rather than to the neck. In fact, parotitis may be suspected because swelling of the glands spreads beyond the angle of the jaw.

The tongue in Phytolacca and Mercurius patients is almost identical; although possibly in some cases with a generally coated tongue, in

Phytolacca the tip of the tongue may be red, in Mercurius there is a general coating all over.

In Phytolacca there is a common tendency for the pain to shoot into the ears on swallowing, whereas in Mercurius the pain is generally in the throat, only occasionally shooting into the ear.

The temperature reaction is slightly different. Instead of the very hot, sweaty state of the Mercurius patient, with shivering if they are uncovered, Phytolacca patients feel hot but also feel shivery without being uncovered.

Patients with a marked aggravation from hot drinks are much more likely to require Phytolacca than Mercurius. Mercurius has the aggravation slightly, Phytolacca acutely.

In Phytolacca the face is very flushed, with a feeling of great heat in the throat and mouth, and patients often say that their tongue feels as if it had been scalded. They always complain of a feeling of fullness in the throat, and an incessant desire to swallow, and yet the act of swallowing is extremely painful. The pain is situated right in the base of the tongue more than in the throat itself, and from there it tends to shoot up into the ears. The discomfort from the throat is very much aggravated by any hot application, hot drinks particularly. There is usually a yellow coating, particularly down the centre of the tongue – very often the edges of the tongue or the tip are quite clear. The tonsillitis may be accompanied by aching pains, usually in the legs or lumbar region, or moving from joint to joint, possibly amounting to a general bruised sensation all over. With these general aching pains the patients are restless. They want to move but they get no relief; rather, there is an aggravation of the pains from movement. The throat appears considerably swollen; it is almost oedematous, particularly the uvula. There may be ulceration of the tonsils, typically a yellow sloughing ulcer on the tonsil, which is extremely sensitive. As a rule, there is more involvement of the right side of the throat than the left. In spite of the general restlessness, these patients almost always complain of giddiness on sitting up or getting out of bed for any reason. They are liable to faint and are always distressed. At first, if undisturbed, they are sluggish. The temperature is high and they are always apprehensive and depressed. In spite of the local aggravation from warmth and hot drinks, they themselves are usually chilly. They feel the cold and they like to be covered up.

They have much the same difficulty in swallowing as in Mercurius, a feeling as if the throat was obstructed. There is not the same degree of salivation in Phytolacca as in Mercurius.

Phytolacca has one very distinctive feature – an acute pain in the base of the tongue when it is protruded. It is an almost diagnostic symptom of Phytolacca if there is any doubt between Phytolacca and Mercurius.

The throats considered so far are all fairly common types. There are one or two others which are not so common, but which give very useful indications for homoeopathic remedies.

Apis

A sore throat which has developed very acutely, which is much aggravated by heat or hot drinks and relieved by cold, and in which any attempt to swallow fluids produces a sensation of acute constriction in the throat with complete inability to swallow, may indicate Apis. The patient feels extremely hot, is very much aggravated by any heat, a hot room, and particularly by radiant heat.

On examination, the throat is very red. In addition to the acute inflammatory appearance there is a very marked oedematous tendency. The whole soft palate, uvula and pillars of the fauces look oedematous, as if they were full of water, and there may be a certain amount of swelling of the tongue also.

As a rule the inflammation starts or is more marked on the right side of the throat, and spreads from there.

These cases respond very well to Apis, prescribed on the oedematous appearance of the throat, accompanied by the marked aggravation from heat, either general or local.

These patients have a high temperature. Incidentally, quite apart from throats, marked oedema is associated with Apis in other conditions as well. Acute angioneurotic oedema will respond well to Apis. Many years ago a woman was seen with angioneurotic oedema which came on suddenly during the night, affecting the whole side from below the neck right down to underneath her costal margin. The condition cleared up almost at once on Apis.

Fish poisoning cases with oedema also respond to Apis, usually in the 200c potency.

Oedema, bright red colour, a burning sensation and an aggravation from warmth are indications for Apis.

Belladonna

Belladonna is needed for acute sore throats which are extremely painful, with a sensation of dryness of the throat and burning pain. It develops very suddenly, with a feeling as if the throat is swelling up, and there is inability to swallow. Any attempt to swallow is attended by violent pain and seems to set up an acute spasm of all the throat muscles. It is accompanied by a very high temperature, a good deal of nervous excitement, and a full bounding pulse, red face and dry skin. On examination, the throat is bright red, very often with small aphthous patches on the tonsils, usually with a dry tongue, slightly coated. There is extreme sensitivity of the throat to touch. These cases clear up very quickly with a few doses of Belladonna, 30c or 200c.

Baptisia

For septic throats the most commonly indicated remedy of all is Baptisia.

The patients are obviously toxic, they look heavy and bloated, they are uncomfortable, the skin is hot and moist, the sweat is offensive, and the mouth is particularly offensive. There is always a very dirty tongue. It may be brownish-yellow and greasy to touch, or it may be brown and dry, or else yellowish with a thick brown streak down the middle. There is an early tendency to ulceration of the tonsils, and the ulcers are dirty-looking. Baptisia is one of the remedies to consider for Vincent's Angina – that is the type of throat. There is always a quantity of very sticky, ropy saliva about the mouth, and particularly the throat. There is always swelling in the neck and round the pillars of the fauces.

The throat itself is dusky in colour, and the patients give the impression of being dusky. They are a bad colour.

Any attempt at swallowing solids is impossible; the patients simply choke, but swallowing fluids sometimes gives a certain degree of comfort.

As a rule these throats are extremely painful. Occasionally one may present with all the general symptoms of the toxic state, offensiveness, the appearance of the tongue, but be almost painless – and yet Baptisia is indicated. It is one of the really severely infected throats, and the cases in which it has been most clearly indicated have often been cases of Vincent's Angina. It is worth remembering that diphtheria and Vincent's Angina may be combined, a very nasty proposition. These cases do best by tackling the Vincent first and the diphtheria afterwards. Given Baptisia to start with, the Vincent's Angina clears in about 24 hours; then treat the diphtheria, which responds very well to Mercurius or Merc. Cy. in most cases and complements the effect of antitoxin.

Two other remedies for septic throats are Lachesis and Hepar. Sulph. They are a very useful contrast, because the Lachesis patient is hot and the Hepar Sulph. patient is cold.

Lachesis

Lachesis patients typically complain that the throat feels swollen and that the fullness extends into the neck, yet on examination there is very little swelling to be seen. Very often they complain that as they fall asleep they have to sit up in bed – they feel as if the throat had completely closed and they are choking.

Lachesis patients with sore throats are always dusky in colour, and look congested. They are very liable to get a pain right through to the base of the skull, extending down the back of the neck, and they complain of the neck being extremely stiff.

In the throat there is always a quantity of very tough mucus which they have great difficulty in clearing. There is a constant desire to swallow, and yet any attempt at swallowing is extremely painful. It is less painful for them to swallow fluids or solids than just to attempt to swallow the saliva. Any attempt at swallowing hot fluids produces an acute spasm in the throat, making swallowing impossible. Hot fluids increase the discomfort in the throat, whereas cold fluids give a degree of relief.

Looking at the throat, some ulceration may be present, but much more commonly there is a very dusky, purplish swelling of the tonsils. And in Lachesis there is a tendency for the trouble to start on the left side, spreading from there to the right.

Lycopodium takes the place of Lachesis for septic throats, just about as painful as the Lachesis ones, but without the aggravation from warm drinks and with an amelioration from warmth. This is particularly true where the trouble starts on the right side instead of the left, and where the patient is not so hot and not so generally congested. But do not prescribe Lycopodium because a condition appears to be right-sided if it has definite Lachesis indications. Lachesis will work in a right-sided inflammation provided the general Lachesis indications are there.

Hepar Sulphuricum

The other remedy frequently indicated for acute septic throats is Hepar Sulph. In Hepar Sulph. the pains in the throat are much more acute and stabbing, in contrast to the feeling of general swelling and choking of Lachesis. Instead of the general toxic state accompanying Lachesis sore throats, Hepar Sulph. patients tend to be much more irritable.

There is the same tendency to early suppuration in the two remedies, but in Hepar Sulph. the patients are always intensely chilly. They want to be covered up, and any draught of air is complained of. They are impatient and very difficult to please.

The Hepar Sulph. throat is always acutely sensitive, and the patients resent examination. There is not the same tendency to glandular enlargement in Hepar Sulph. as there is in Lachesis.

In addition to their chilliness, in Hepar Sulph. there is always a tendency to sweat, particularly about the head. It is often a cold sweat, whereas in Lachesis the skin is hot and sticky.

As a rule, in Hepar Sulph. associated with the acute sore throat, patients develop a very irritable cough – a sort of barking cough, which is very distressing to the throat.

Chapter 4

Respiratory Conditions

COLDS

Gelsemium and Eupatorium
There are two outstanding remedies in the Materia Medica for the usual types of cold, and these are Gelsemium and Eupatorium. The cold which requires either Gels. or Eupatorium is the typical feverish one. The patients say they have a feverish cold, a slight headache, they feel cold and ache, they shiver in the cold air, the shivers going up and down the spine, their nose becomes obstructed in a hot room, and they feel unwell generally. That is the typical Gels. cold. If it progresses further, and instead of just feeling unwell they are aching from head to toe, if it is painful to move and there are signs of a catarrhal cold with an increased feeling of weariness, and a definitely increased sensitiveness to change of temperature – that is the typical Eupatorium. These two remedies will cover the majority of the ordinary feverish colds.

Allium Cepa
There are two outstanding remedies for the ordinary streaming cold in the head. The commonest is Allium Cepa. The patients have a profuse watery nasal discharge with a feeling of heat and burning in the nose, a tendency to excoriation of the upper lip, maybe a slight rise of temperature, but with very little in the way of general symptoms. If it has been untreated for 48 hours or so it usually sets up a laryngeal irritation with a very sensitive larynx. There is excoriation of the upper lip and apparently excoriation of the larynx as well. That is the later stage of the ordinary Allium Cepa acute coryza, and is much the most common.

Euphrasia
The other type is one in which there is a similarly profuse nasal discharge, but where the discharge is not excoriating and is accom-

panied by a good deal of conjunctivitis, congestion of the eyes, a certain amount of photophobia and redness of the eyelids. In other words, the lachrymal discharge is irritating but the nasal discharge is not. That case responds to Euphrasia.

Arsenicum Album
Occasionally a patient appears as a fairly typical Allium Cepa patient; there is the excoriating, burning, nasal discharge, but there is rather more temperature, rather more chilliness and the burning tends to extend back into the fauces. There is a certain amount of post-nasal discharge which is again hot and burning, accompanied by thirst and general chilliness. That case usually responds to a few doses of Arsenicum Album in a low potency.

Mercurius
In a patient where the cold starts with irritation in the throat, either pain or burning in the tonsillar region with difficulty in swallowing, a feeling of fullness and a few hours later they have a pouring coryza, a few doses of Mercurius are usually indicated.

It is impossible to cover the whole Materia Medica that applies to colds. These above are the most common useful remedies in general practice.

BRONCHITIS

Moving a little further down the respiratory tract and considering acute bronchitis, there are three remedies which will help greatly in treating the average case.

A child starting an attack of acute bronchitis, with rapidly increasing mucus secretion, very distressing cough, an obvious temperature and râles all over the chest, will almost always respond to Ipecacuanha. If it is a little more severe, the child obviously more ill, the râles more extensive in the chest, the child becoming rather cyanotic, and the tongue definitely coated, instead of Ipecacuanha give Antimonium Tart. These two remedies will deal with most cases of acute bronchitis in the child.

Acute bronchitis in the adult; the patient who comes every winter with an acute bronchitis, which is really only an aggravation of his chronic bronchitis, will be relieved by Ammonium Carb. almost every time. There is often a certain amount of arterial sclerosis, a certain amount of emphysema and a sticky sputum, the patients getting a profuse, watery sputum, as well as a tough sputum which they cannot expel due to the chronic condition. These patients will respond well to Ammonium Carb. It diminishes their sputum, relieves their heart and loosens their cough. Several doses of the 30c potency should be given.

There are three remedies to consider when dealing with the child who has a dry wheezing distressing cough, depending very largely on the time of day at which they are most distressed. If the paroxysm of coughing begins early in the evening with a dry chest, a few doses of Aconite will relieve it. If the main distress is round about the early hours of the morning, midnight to 2, 3 or 4 a.m., a few doses of Spongia will alleviate. If there is relief from either Aconite or Spongia but it does not hold them, or if the cough begins later in the night – after 4 a.m. – or is mainly troublesome in the day, then Hepar Sulph. is the main standby.

The tiresome, irritating, tickling cough of tracheitis is usually controlled by Drosera. An acute feverish tracheitis that has spread downwards from the throat will usually respond to Allium Cepa.

PNEUMONIA

Bryonia and Phosphorus

For the treatment of pneumonias there are two remedies much more commonly indicated than any others, Bryonia and Phosphorus. The main distinguishing features between Bryonia and Phosphorus pneumonias are that Bryonia patients are more toxic, heavy and slightly cyanotic. They dislike being disturbed, usually have a very painful cough, with a good deal of pain in the chest which is relieved by pressure – either lying on the affected side, or by holding the side when coughing. The patients have a white-coated tongue and are thirsty for fairly large quantities of cold water. Not infrequently the paroxysms of coughing are relieved by hot drinks, which is not what the patients feel they want. It does not matter which lung is involved; it is probably more commonly indicated in the right side, but Bryonia will act equally well in a left-sided pneumonia.

In the Phosphorus pneumonias the patients are more anxious, much more awake, flushed, not cyanotic, and are as thirsty as the Bryonia patients, often for ice-cold drinks. But they do not have nearly such a coated tongue, dislike any pressure on the affected area, and tend to lie on the unaffected side. Again it does not matter what area of the lung is involved, although it is probably more commonly the lower lobe that is involved in a Phosphorus pneumonia.

The probability is that the Bryonia pneumonia has developed rather more slowly, and the Phosphorus pneumonia has come on fairly acutely.

POST-INFLUENZAL COMPLICATIONS AND SEQUELAE

Probably the most common sequela of influenza is a persisting infection of one or other of the accessory nasal sinuses, antrum, ethmoidal cells or frontal sinus. Next in frequency is persistent catarrh of the eustachian tube and middle ear. These two complications not infrequently occur at the same time.

Another very common and trying result of an influenzal attack is persistent trouble in the respiratory tract, showing itself as an obstinate, distressing and often intractable cough.

Less commonly, but still quite frequently, are cases in which the digestive system seems to have been upset, with symptoms suggestive of a subacute gastritis, gastro-duodenitis, or even cholecystitis or hepatitis.

The most common general sequelae are persistent weakness and nervous depression.

As a rule, where prescribing for the acute attack has been accurate such trials are not met with, but even with the best endeavours, they do still occur.

Taking the sequelae in a little more detail; first the accessory sinuses and naso-pharynx, the remedies most frequently indicated are Kali Bich. and Silica.

Kali Bichromicum
In patients needing Kali Bich. there has been a persistence of sticky discharge, associated with pain or a sense of fullness, or pressure over the frontal sinuses or the antra, and usually a sense of obstruction at the bridge of the nose. These post-influenzal Kali Bich. patients are always classical examples of post-influenzal debility, and their symptoms are acutely aggravated in cold damp weather and better in a warm bed. If they complain of sharp, pressing pain over the affected sinus, that is a confirmatory symptom of great value.

Silica

Contrast that picture with the one presented by Silica. At first sight the two appear to be almost identical. Both show signs of general debility, both show aggravation in cold damp weather, and in both there is a complaint of fullness or pressure in the affected sinus. In Kali Bich. this involvement is accompanied by profuse discharge, while in Silica there is no discharge and a steadily increasing tension in the affected sinus.

Pulsatilla

There is a different type of case in which the symptoms of the patient are aggravated by heat, close rooms or a stuffy atmosphere, suggestive of Pulsatilla. There is not so much active involvement of the sinuses in Pulsatilla, but the patient complains that the nose is blocked, often very marked on waking in the morning and getting worse again towards evening, and especially in a warm room. It is better in the open air. This is not infrequently associated with a very unpleasant odour of which the patient is acutely conscious.

Pulsatilla, though seldom indicated for involvement of the sinuses, is quite often indicated in catarrhal involvement of the ear in cases which may go on to acute otitis media with sharp stabbing pains in the ear.

Mercurius and Kali Iodatum

Where there is involvement of the sinuses in patients who are sensitive to heat, enquire for indications suggesting either Mercurius or Kali Iod. Both have acute involvement of the sinuses with acute pain. In Mercurius the patient has marked aggravation from radiant heat, associated with a sense of fullness in the affected sinus, a tendency to perspire and violent pains. The Mercurius patient is very sensitive to draughts and will exhibit the typical pale flabby indented tongue of Mercurius.

When dealing with a case showing such acute sensitiveness to draughts it is always worth while to remember that a case of that kind, improving but not cured by Mercurius, may later be helped by Hepar Sulph.

In Kali Iod. patients there may be trouble in any of the sinuses, with an acute sense of tightness, often accompanied by stabbing pains. There is marked aggravation in a warm room, with a sense of general weariness, and the patient is much better walking about in the open air. It is more frequently indicated in infections of the frontal, sphenoid or ethmoid sinuses rather than the antra.

Pyrogen
When the deeper sinuses are involved, Pyrogen may be indicated. There is usually a marked toxaemia with general aching, slight attacks of shivering alternating with a feeling of heat, and a pulse temperature discrepancy.

Hydrastis
Post-influenzal coughs can be particularly troublesome. There are the cases in which the patient complains of rawness and irritation of the naso-pharynx, with a bad cough aggravated by talking or smoking and which is often worrying at night. For this condition Hydrastis is the greatest help, especially for cases with a reddened congested pharynx and streaks of yellow muco-pus trickling down from the posterior nares.

Alumina
Alumina is another remedy increasingly indicated in such cases of persistent pharyngitis. There is not nearly so much secretion, in fact the pharynx often has a somewhat dry appearance. The patients complain of its being very sensitive and sore, with sticking pains. Periodically there seems to be an accumulation of ropy mucus which must be expectorated, and this is accompanied by a feeling of soreness in the larynx and trachea, with a hacking cough.

Two other medicines frequently indicated are Nux Vomica and Conium.

Nux Vomica
Indications helpful in the Nux Vomica patient are acute irritation in one or other tonsillar region, setting up a violent cough which continues until there is the expectoration of some mucus or muco-purulent sputum, after which they have peace for a time. This, when associated with a tendency to nasal congestion in a hot room, and accompanied by some gastric acidity, is a strong indication for Nux Vomica.

Conium
There appears to be a close similarity in Conium, in that the patient has a violent paroxysmal cough due to irritation in the throat. The irritation, however, is in the pharynx or larynx rather than in the tonsillar region. It is liable to come on when the patient is lying in bed or on taking a deep breath. It is unaccompanied by the heartburn met with in Nux Vomica. Though the patient may say he has to sit up and

cough to clear the irritation, this does not mean, as in Nux Vomica, that there is relief immediately on the expectoration of some sputum.

LARYNGITIS AND TRACHEITIS

Further down the respiratory tract, the cases with persistent irritation in the larynx and trachea must be considered. With their clear-cut indications of irritation at the level of the supra-sternal notch and their aggravation from change of temperature, Phosphorus or Rumex immediately come to mind, and they do cover a large number of cases. The next most frequently indicated remedy is Carbo Veg. for people who are below par generally. Their colds do not clear and the inflammation extends to the larynx and trachea. They become husky, particularly in the evening. They get attacks of most exhausting cough, almost like whooping cough, in which they become red in the face and damp with sweat, gasping for air, and after which they are exhausted. The larynx feels raw and is often tender to touch. These are indications for Carbo Veg.

Never think of whooping cough without considering Drosera. Drosera is occasionally called for in post-influenzal coughs which come on after eating or drinking, or are liable to be very troublesome on lying down at night or round 3 a.m., and are of this violent spasmodic nature with a most distressing irritation in the larynx.

Then never think of spasmodic coughs without recalling Hepar Sulph. and Spongia. Hepar Sulph. with its hypersensitiveness to any cold air or becoming cold, with rattling in the chest. And Spongia with its cough coming on just after midnight, a dry cough, accompanied by anxiety, cardiac oppression, and aggravation in a warm room but amelioration from warm drinks.

One of the commoner laryngeal troubles which persist is hoarseness. Here, consideration of a fresh group of remedies is required in addition to those already mentioned. Carbo Veg. and Phosphorus are often needed, but even more frequently there are indications for Causticum. The patient complains of hoarseness in the morning which usually improves during the day. There is violent coughing in an endeavour to clear the mucus from the respiratory tract and patients often say that they cannot cough deeply enough to clear it, but if they can expectorate the voice improves. The attacks of coughing may be relieved by a drink of cold water, and the patient may have loss of urinary control during the violent attacks of coughing. This hoarseness, if accompanied by the general aching tiredness of the post-influenza period, especially if symptoms are worse in cold dry weather, is almost certain to respond to Causticum.

Causticum is similar to Arum Triphyllum, which has all the symptoms of an ordinary influenza, especially the aching in the bones. As a rule, the patient will say that the condition started with a very excoriating nasal discharge accompanied by intense irritation in the nose, most marked on the left side. This was followed by a raw feeling behind the sternum with loss of voice, the peculiarity being the ability to speak on either a higher or lower note than usual, progressing to complete loss of voice.

In other cases where the voice is lost with use there may be indications for Rhus Tox. The patients have the dry tormenting cough, coming in paroxysms, with aching pains all round the ribs, and the general mental and physical restlessness of Rhus Tox.

It is not practicable to discuss all the possible remedies which may be required in cases showing persistent chest trouble. However, apart from the use of a nosode, the remedies likely to be indicated are Silica, Phosphorus, Carbo Veg., Calcarea Carb., Lycopodium, Sulphur and Pulsatilla in the chronic and Kreosote, Sanguinaria, Senega, Kali Carb. and Antimonium Tart. in the more acute stages.

DIGESTIVE SEQUELAE

Kali Bichromicum

The common digestive sequelae of influenzal attacks are usually catarrhal in nature, and the remedy most commonly indicated in these cases is Kali Bich. The symptoms are usually somewhat vague, such as weakness of digestion and being upset by the simplest of foods. The disturbances are of two kinds, either distension and obstructed flatus in stomach and bowel with repletion after the smallest meal, or sharp pains. The pains are cutting or burning in character with soreness and tenderness in the epigastrium, usually towards the left in a small spot — rather suggestive of a gastric ulcer — coming on usually after 1 a.m., between 1 a.m. and 3 a.m. There is often a sense of emptiness with aversion to food, and a marked aggravation from starchy food, especially potatoes. X-ray may reveal a marked excess of mucus, increased gastric mobility and exaggeration of the normal pattern of the mucous membrane. With such symptoms, consider the possibility of Kali Bich., but the symptomatology suggests the possibility of several other remedies being required: Lycopodium, for instance with its flatulence, empty feeling and repletion after a small meal. The patient would have the typical Lycopodium make-up of the tired, thin, wrinkled, chronic dyspeptic, aggravated by cold drinks and relieved by warm, and sensitive to beer, coffee and fruit. China presents a very similar picture with its feeling of hunger yet aversion to food, its acute flatulent distension and its general debility. China is also indicated for the extremely sensitive nervous patient liable to attacks of diarrhoea after a meal, upset by fruit, fish and particularly wine, and likely to have violent attacks of colic coming on at midnight. In cases with extreme flatulent distension after any food, Carbo Veg. is needed. In Carbo Veg. there is outstanding relief from eructation: without this, Carbo Veg. is not indicated, no matter how suggestive the other symptoms may be.

Bryonia

In the digestive complications of influenza, as opposed to the sequelae, the drug most frequently indicated is Bryonia. This has a classical picture of acute gastritis, with extreme abdominal sensitivity, intense nausea, aggravated by any movement, better after eructations and with relief from hot drinks. This complication yields very readily to Bryonia.

Antimonium Crudum

Antimonium Crudum is indicated in those cases in which the catarrhal symptoms have persisted with a tendency for the nose to be blocked up in the evening in a warm room, and with digestive symptoms. There is a thickly-coated white tongue, and the patient complains of a constant sensation of fullness and heaviness in the stomach, as if they had overeaten. There is a feeling of acute distenstion though there is no swelling of the abdomen, and aversion to the thought or smell of all food. All digestive symptoms are greatly aggravated by becoming cold or by drinking anything sour.

DEPRESSION

Aurum Metallicum

Depression is a common sequela of influenza. The first remedy which immediately comes to mind is Aurum, with its acute depression and feeling that everything is wrong, looking on the black side of everything, expecting trouble and looking for it. The patients are obstinate, irritable and very easily annoyed. They have flushes of heat and are better in the open air, frequently they suffer from palpitation and often have slight exophthalmos. They may have oedema of the ankles. Not infrequently Aurum is indicated in cases of post-influenzal arthritis, with pains which are worse at night compelling the patient to get out of bed and move about.

Pulsatilla
Another type of depression usually responds to Pulsatilla. Here there is the same sensitivity to heat and a somewhat similar depressed state, where the patient tends to be miserable and sits about saying nothing, but the picture is in essence very different. In Pulsatilla the patients are sensitive. There are liable to be tears and irritation. They feel that they are being misunderstood or slighted in some way, and hate to be interrupted in what they are doing. Often they think that no one realises how ill they feel and they are miserable about it. They are restless and better when moving about and occupied. They are hot-blooded and hate a lot of clothing, are difficult to feed and complain of feeling full up hours after a meal.

Silica
Silica is another remedy which may be required for post-influenzal depression. The patients are depressed because they feel incompetent, that they cannot cope with life and especially with the problems of the moment, although in reality they manage perfectly well. They are shy and retiring, and liable to be irritable when aroused. After an attack of influenza there may be persistent enlargement of the cervical glands. They feel tired and suffer from headaches spreading over from the back of the head, accompanied by dampness of the forehead and extreme sensitiveness of the head to cold air. These patients are aggravated by cold and becoming cold, but they cannot stand extremes of either heat or cold.

EXHAUSTION

For post-influenzal nervous exhaustion there are three remedies of the greatest value, namely, Picric Acid, Phosphoric Acid and Cocculus Indicus. In all of them there is the same feeling of weariness and inability to sustain any mental effort.

Picric Acid

The main complaint in Picric Acid is that any attempt at mental application produces a violent headache, accompanied by trembling, faintness, numbness and extreme lassitude. The patients feel they simply must lie down. They become indifferent and do not want to do anything. Typically they are useless during the day and are much better during the evening. They are sensitive to heat and are often relieved by bathing the head with cold water. Any physical exertion is followed by a feeling of complete exhaustion.

Phosphoric Acid

The Phosphoric Acid picture is somewhat different. Here there is a state of torpor associated with the mental weariness. The patients do not want to talk, they feel so tired. They suffer from headaches with a sense of pressure on the top of the head, which is brought on by any exertion. They complain of cold extremities and are liable to have cold damp hands. They are sensitive to cold, though they cannot stand a stuffy room. Frequently they complain of acute skin irritation on any part of the body. Often they say that since influenza their hair has been falling out. They may complain of giddiness and a sensation of floating. Usually Phosphoric Acid patients suffer from indigestion with a sense of the food taking hours to digest, and are liable to attacks of diarrhoea, which surprisingly seem to brighten them up. They quite often complain of bone pains, described as if the bones were being scraped.

Cocculus Indicus

Lastly there is Cocculus Indicus. The typical picture is that of mental and physical prostration. All the reactions are slowed down and convalescence is correspondingly slow. The patients cannot be hurried, they want a long time to do everything, all the movements are slow. There is a tendency to incoordination and they are liable to drop things, and complain of sudden jerking of the limbs. They are liable to suffer from violent headaches with nausea and vomiting. These may be brought on by any form of travelling, by car, boat, train or aeroplane. They suffer from great weakness in the knees and back, often with a sense of stiffness in the joints and a feeling of being almost paralysed, frequently coupled with a feeling of numbness. They are very sensitive to noise, jarring, or any sudden movement. The appetite is practically lost and there may be an acute aversion even to the thought of food. They suffer from sleeplessness and are prostrated by any loss of sleep.

Chapter 5

Heart Conditions

The simplest way to group cardiac emergencies from a remedy point of view is to look at them under three headings: 1) Acute cardiac failure, 2) Gradual cardiac failure with a tendency to dilatation, and 3) Acute cardiac angina.

ACUTE CARDIAC FAILURE

For acute cardiac failure, most cases require one of four remedies. These are Arsenicum Alb., Antimony Tart., Carbo Veg. and Oxalic Acid. There are various points which help in the selection of these individual remedies and it is not difficult to distinguish between them.

Arsenicum Album
Arsenicum Alb. patients demonstrate the typical Arsenicum Alb. mental distress, with extreme fear, extreme anxiety, and mental and physical restlessness. They have constant thirst, with a desire for small sips of cold water.

The main complaint is a feeling of extreme cardiac pressure, a feeling of great weight or constriction of the chest. At the same time the patients feel as if they cannot get enough air into the lungs and that they are going to die.

As a rule Arsenicum Alb. patients are cold, they feel cold, though they may complain of some burning pain in the chest.

In appearance they always look extremely anxious. They are grey, their lips are rather pale, maybe a little cyanotic, and they are very dangerously ill. They often have a peculiar pinched, wrinkled, grey appearance.

As a rule there is a history that the attack has developed quite suddenly, and the response to Arsenicum Alb. should be equally quick. The first response is a diminution of the patient's mental anxiety and extreme fear, the restlessness begins to subside, and they begin to feel a little warmer.

Arsenicum Alb. seems to act very much like a temporary cardiac stimulant, and in the majority of these cases it is necessary to repeat the dose frequently and to give it in a high potency.

There is a very important practical point in connection with these cases. A patient has responded well to Arsenicum Alb., his condition has improved and then in 3, 4 or 6 hours he has a relapse. If Arsenicum Alb. is repeated the patient does not improve a second time. To avoid this it is necessary to prescribe a second remedy within 4–6 hours of the primary collapse, while the patient is still responding to the Arsenicum Alb. This should prevent the secondary collapse. This seems to be one of the very few instances which appears to ride right across the dictum that so long as the patient is improving, continue with the same remedy. In these acute Arsenicum Alb. cases, if the patient improves, a second remedy needs to be prescribed within 2–3 hours.

The remedies which frequently follow Arsenicum Alb. in the reactive stage are Phosphorus or Sulphur, but that is by no means constant. One can easily picture that grey, pinched, anxious Arsenicum Alb. patient responding, getting a little warmer, a little less grey, a little less pinched and drawn, a little less anxious and restless and becoming a typical Phosphorus patient. Equally one can see them going to the other extreme, where they are too hot, with irregular waves of heat and cold, tending to push the blankets off, with air hunger and requiring Sulphur.

These are the two commonest remedies, but one other that can be helpful following Arsenicum Alb. is Carbo Veg. Here the air hunger persists and the patient has to sit up to get comfortable, he has troublesome flatulence, the extremities are very cold, but the thirst is subsiding. The patient is slightly cyanosed, perspiring and has a craving for fresh air, moving fresh air, and asks to be fanned. With these symptoms Carbo Veg. is indicated.

Antimonium Tartrate

Antimonium Tart. patients present a somewhat similar picture to Arsenicum Alb., but there are clear points of difference. Antimonium Tart. have a greater tendency towards cyanosis than Arsenicum Alb. This may involve the whole of the extremities or it may be confined to the nails.

There is never the same kind of mental anxiety in Antimonium Tart. They are more exhausted, much more hopeless, more depressed. They are never quite as restless and never quite so pale as Arsenicum Alb. They are not thirsty, and drinking seems to increase the patient's distress.

Another contrast is that Antimonium Tart. are very much aggravated by heat, and especially by a stuffy atmosphere. As a contrast between Antimonium Tart. and Carbo Veg., Antimonium Tart. patients do not like a stream of air circulating round them; they want the room fresh, but they like the air to be still.

In most of these Antimonium Tart. cases there is an early tendency to oedema of the lower extremities.

Another indication for Antimonium Tart. is that practically all these patients have a very white thickly-coated tongue, with a rather sticky, uncomfortable mouth.

They have a feeling of fullness in the chest, rather than the feeling of acute pressure found in Arsenicum Alb. Frequently, generalised, diffuse râles are present in the lower part of the lungs on both sides.

In contrast to the Arsenicum Alb. patient with collapse after a cardiac crisis, patients responding to Antimonium Tart. will continue to improve without the need of a follow-up remedy as is necessary in Arsenicum Alb.

Carbo Vegetabilis
Carbo Veg. patients present the classical picture of collapse. They have the cold clammy skin, are mentally dull and confused, and have no very clear idea of their surroundings or what is happening to them. They have the most intense air hunger, and in spite of their cold clammy extremities want the air blowing on them. They cannot bear to have the bedclothes round their necks and they benefit from oxygen.

They are much paler than the Antimonium Tart. patients; the lips tend to be pale rather than cyanotic.

Like the Antimonium Tart. patients, any attempt to eat or drink tends to increase their distress, and they have none of the Arsenicum Alb. thirst.

An apparent contradiction in Carbo Veg. patients is that, in spite of their desire to be uncovered and their intolerance of the blankets round the upper part of the neck or chest, they complain of ice-cold extremities. They feel as if the legs are just lumps of ice and they cannot get them warm at all.

Once the patient is responding to Carbo Veg. – perspiring less, the surface becoming warmer and the distress less acute – it is wise then to look for a second remedy in case of need, because some Carbo Veg.

patients relapse although many of them make a complete recovery on Carbo Veg. Often when the patient has made some improvement after the administration of Carbo Veg., the follow-up remedy will be found to be Sulphur, although Kali Carb. should always be considered.

Oxalic Acid

The last of these remedies for acute cardiac failure is Oxalic Acid. Oxalic Acid has one or two very outstanding symptoms which are often met with in cases of collapse, and which are a great help in the selection of the remedy.

First, the patients always complain of a feeling of the most intense exhaustion. Associated with that exhaustion there is usually a sensation of numbness. They very often say that their legs and feet feel numb and paralysed, or they feel as if they had no legs at all.

The skin surface is about as cold and clammy as it is in Carbo Veg. but Oxalic Acid patients have a peculiar mottled cyanosis not present in the other remedies. The fingertips and finger and toe nails will be cyanotic but in addition, the patients have a peculiar mottled appearance of the hands and feet which is quite distinctive to Oxalic Acid. This mottled cyanotic condition also occurs on the face, usually over the malar bones.

These patients, in contrast to Arsenicum Alb., want to keep absolutely still; movement of any kind increases their distress.

In addition to their general distress, most Oxalic Acid patients complain of sharp pains in the chest. The pain is not typical anginal pain; it is a sharp pricking pain which usually comes through from the back and extends up the left side of the sternum towards the clavicle, or down the left side of the sternum into the epigastrium.

GRADUAL CARDIAC FAILURE WITH A TENDENCY TO DILATATION

Now to consider cases where the heart is gradually failing, beginning to dilate, becoming slightly irregular, and the patients are obviously going downhill. In many of these patients with early cardiac failure, the heart improves and the dilatation disappears in response to ordinary routine prescribing, and it is not necessary to consider the cardiac symptoms particularly. The patients respond to the remedy for their general symptoms. For instance, quite frequently in pneumonia – a severe pneumonia, with a failing heart, with dilatation – after the administration of Lycopodium, the pulse steadies and the dilatation of the heart disappears. This occurs in all acute illnesses where the patient is responding to the particular remedy indicated. However, there are cases in which the patient improves but the cardiac failure does not respond to the individual remedy, and here it is necessary to prescribe for the cardiac failure.

These patients most readily respond to the Snake remedies, especially Lachesis and Naja, less commonly to the plants Lycopus and Laurocerasus.

It is very difficult to distinguish one Snake remedy from another for such conditions. In appearance the patients are all very similar, but much the most commonly indicated are Lachesis and Naja.

Lachesis and Naja
The Lachesis picture is typical of all the Snake remedies, but there are a few indications which make Naja the choice in preference to Lachesis.

All patients for whom the Snake remedies are indicated have a cyanosed, bloated appearance. They all complain of a feeling of tightness or constriction in the chest, more commonly in the upper part of the chest, and they are all intolerant of any weight or pressure of the bedclothes or any tight clothing around the upper part of the chest or the neck. All are sensitive to heat, they feel hot and they dislike a hot stuffy room. They all have a marked aggravation after sleep. They get acute suffocative attacks when they fall asleep, and they wake up in increased distress.

All of these patients in their cardiac distress have a marked aggravation from being turned over on the left side. All of them have a very marked tremor. And most of them, as they get worse, become mentally dull and confused, and often tend to become difficult and suspicious.

If these were all the symptoms, Lachesis would be the indicated remedy. A certain number of patients have acute stitching pains which go right through the chest from the precordium to the region of the scapula, associated with numbness, particularly in the left arm and hand. These are the indications for Naja in preference to Lachesis.

If the pain – stitching pain – is more marked, Naja is indicated. If the feeling of constriction is more marked, give Lachesis. Their general symptoms are identical. Possibly Naja patients are a little less congested, less bloated looking and a little paler than Lachesis patients, but that is not very striking.

Apart from the Snake remedies there are two others which are very useful in these conditions, Lycopus and Laurocerasus.

Lycopus

Indications for Lycopus may occur in patients with early signs of heart failure. Their pulse is slightly irregular and the heart beginning to dilate. The patients tend to be pale rather than cyanotic, and they are always restless.

The outstanding symptoms of Lycopus cases is that the patients complain of a tumultuous sensation in the cardiac region. Their heart-beat is completely irregular, and they experience a feeling of intense throbbing extending up into the neck and head. The tumultuous sensation in the chest is usually accompanied by a desire to cough.

Another symptom which distinguishes Lycopus patients is that their discomfort is greatly increased by turning over on to the right side – a contrast with the patients needing Snake remedies, whose cardiac discomfort is worse turning on to the left side.

Lastly, Lycopus patients have an intense dislike of any food, and particularly the smell of food.

Laurocerasus

The Laurocerasus patient presents a definite picture, and the easiest way to remember it is to recall the appearance presented by a con-genital heart patient of about 16 to 18 years of age. Think of the peculiar bluish-red complexion, clubbed fingers, which are rather congested, and the peculiar bluish appearance – almost like ripe grapes – of the lips. That underlying colour is associated with Laurocerasus.

These patients always suffer from extreme dyspnoea, which is nearly Cheyne Stokes in character. They take a sudden gasping breath, then two or three long breaths, then the breathing gets gradually shallower, then a pause, followed by two or three gasps, and this pattern of breathing continues. This dyspnoea gets very much worse if the patients sit upright. They are easier in a semi-recumbent position.

There is a marked tendency to the early development of hypostatic pneumonia in such cases, and once this has appeared, the cough is more troublesome unless they are reasonably supported. When lying down the cough is worse, yet sitting upright produces a feeling of extreme constriction of the chest, so that semi-recumbent is the position of choice.

These patients are always cold; they feel cold to touch and want to be kept warm, and any movement or exertion causes an acute aggravation.

Two other remedies are of great value in treating heart conditions, namely Crataegus Oxyacantha and Latrodectus Mactans.

Crataegus Oxyacantha

Crataegus is of the greatest value in myocardial degeneration with a steadily failing heart. In such a condition there will be the usual accompanying symptoms, increasing pulse rate, signs of pulmonary congestion, a certain amount of oedema, slight cyanosis and aggravation from any exertion.

In such a condition, Crataegus in low potency may produce a dramatic effect and a considerable amount of recovery in the apparently irreparably damaged heart. Give Crataegus 3x every 3 to 4 hours for several weeks.

Latrodectus Mactans

The indications for Latrodectus are also in cases of cardiac failure such as those with a definite valvular lesion.

As in Crataegus, there are the usual physical signs of a failing heart, but Latrodectus patients are in addition always very irritable. They complain of numbness of the left hand and arm, and they usually have precordial pain which may be of any degree of severity.

These patients will get great relief from the administration of Latrodectus 12c or 30c, given at short intervals, say every 2 to 4 hours, for 24 hours, and then repeated only when necessary.

ACUTE CARDIAC ANGINA

Patients with true or pseudo-angina often give cause for anxiety, but there are a few homoeopathic remedies which give great relief to many of them.

Aconite

The outstanding characteristic of the majority of patients in their first attack of angina pectoris is an overwhelming fear. The patient is certain he is going to die and that he is going to die very speedily, and he is terrified. He is quite unable to keep still, and yet any movement seems to aggravate his distress. In a patient with these symptoms, a dose of Aconite in a high potency will give relief almost instantly.

The patient may have a similar attack at a later date, and the anxiety, the distress and the fear are not so marked because he has recovered from a previous attack, and Aconite may give no relief at all. In the first attack, when the patient is quite certain he is going to die, Aconite relieves the symptoms straight away, but it has no effect in a second or later attack. In the later attacks of angina pectoris, Cactus is the remedy most likely to give relief.

Cactus

Cactus patients have a good deal of anxiety and fear, but it is quite different from that of Aconite patients. It is not a fear that the immediate attack will kill him, it is more a conviction that he has an absolutely incurable condition which will eventually be fatal.

Another point is the type of the actual distress of which the Cactus patient complains. He feels as if he has a tight band round the chest which is gradually becoming tighter and tighter, and that if this tightness does not let up soon the heart will be unable to function. That feeling of increasing tension gives the Cactus indication.

In addition to the constriction, there may be stabbing, radiating pains from the precordium, but they are not so characteristic of Cactus as the intense feeling of constriction. This is, of course, exactly how the majority of patients with angina pectoris describe their pain.

In these acute conditions, give the remedy in a high potency, because it acts much more quickly and the patient needs relief as quickly as possible.

Arsenicum Album

Occasionally a patient experiences an attack of angina with very similar constricting pain, not quite as intense as in a Cactus patient where the constricting pain seems to dominate the whole picture, but still a feeling of constriction. The patient has been unwell for some time. He is pale, rather anxious and worried, and feels cold, and the feeling of constriction in the chest is accompanied by a rather acute, distressing, burning sensation. These patients respond very well to a dose of Arsenicum Alb.

Iodum

Other patients may complain of very much the same sensation, but the feeling of constriction, the feeling of tension, is described as being actually in the heart itself rather than involving the whole of the side of the chest.

The patients are just about as anxious as Arsenicum Alb. – but instead of the intense coldness of Arsenicum Alb. they are uncomfortable in heat and in a stuffy atmosphere. They are about as restless, but instead of the pale, drawn appearance of Arsenicum Alb., they tend to be rather flushed and, as a rule, are dark-haired, dark-complexioned people. They are usually underweight, in spite of the fact that they often have an appetite above the average. These cases respond exceedingly well to Iodum.

Spongia

Yet another type of case is one in which the complaint, instead of being constriction, is of a sensation of progressive swelling in the heart region. The patients feel as if the heart is swelling more and more and will finally burst, and the sensation of fullness spreads up into the neck.

This sensation of fullness and swelling is very much aggravated by lying down, when the patients feel as if they will choke, and it is accompanied by acute pain.

The patients are chilly, and any draught of air increases their distress. In addition to their discomfort in the chest, they usually complain of numbness, particularly of the left arm and hand, or numbness of the hand without any involvement of the arm. Not infrequently they also complain of numbness of the lower extremities.

As a rule, the face and neck look congested, they do not have the pale, drawn wrinkled appearance of Arsenicum Alb. patients. These cases respond well to Spongia.

Spigelia

Another useful remedy for patients who do not have the typical anginal constriction, but the pseudo-anginal stabbing, radiating pains – sharp, stabbing pains starting in the precordium, spreading up into the neck, maybe across into the right side or down the left arm. These shooting pains may be followed by numbness involving the whole affected area, and as a rule, the pain is a little eased by turning over on to the right side.

Accompanying the stabbing pains there is a degree of hyperaesthesia over the precordium. Any movement aggravates the pain, or brings on a violent attack. These patients respond to Spigelia.

Lilium Tigrinum

There is a condition which is not a true angina but which is met with in hysterical women. No cardiac lesion is demonstrable, but the patients will produce a symptom picture which is difficult to distinguish from a true anginal attack. They have marked stabbing, radiating pains, often an intense hyperaesthesia of the chest wall. They are very depressed and frightened, and they are intensely irritable. They are sensitive to heat, and their distress is aggravated by any movement. In addition to their stabbing pains, they have the anginal sense of constriction, tightness of the chest wall.

If these patients also have a pelvic lesion or a history of having had some gynaecological complaint, they will respond to Lilium Tig.

Chapter 6

The Gastrointestinal Tract

DYSPEPSIA

The ordinary dyspeptic patient seen in the surgery has either an acute attack of indigestion following some indiscretion in diet, or chronic dyspepsia and chronic constipation.

Consider the acute attack. The patients fall quite easily into one of two classes. First, the adult who has been out, eaten and drunk too much, and comes to the surgery next morning feeling indisposed, probably with a slight headache, and very little inclination for breakfast. This type will respond in the majority of instances to a few doses of Nux Vomica in a low potency.

The other type of acute digestive upset is met with more commonly in the child. The child who has been out to a party, eaten too many cakes and ices, been vomiting all night, and is brought in next morning pale, irritable and tired. In the majority of cases all the child needs is a dose of Pulsatilla in either the 6c or 30c potency.

The next type of dyspeptic disturbance is the tired out, weary patient with chronic flatulence. There are mainly two types. There is the thin, nervous patient whose digestive upset has followed some minor acute illness, who has chronic indigestion, a good deal of flatulence, and is rather chilly and irritable. A few doses of China in a low potency will usually clear the symptoms.

In contrast there is the heavy, sluggish, fat, lethargic type with a tendency to eat too much starchy food, a tendency to flatulence and a feeling of fullness and discomfort round the waist. A few doses of Carbo Veg. puts that temporary indiscretion right.

Patients must be considered as individuals. These are broad outlines. Each of these remedies may be used as a heading for a number of others which are complementary. Include with the Nux Vomica patients all the nervy, excitable people who are upset by over-rich food. They may require Nux Vomica, Lycopodium, Ignatia, Arsenicum Alb.

or Phosphorus. All patients of that type are upset by similar things, and Nux Vomica can be put at the head of the group, but the others must be considered.

In children – Pulsatilla, Argentum Nit. and Calcarea Carb. are all liable to be upset in similar circumstances, but Pulsatilla is much the most commonly indicated member of the group.

Another group is the emaciated China type. A similar type of patient may need Sepia, Natrum Mur., Natrum Carb. and occasionally Lycopodium.

In the Carbo Veg. group they may require Graphites, Anacardium, Calcarea Carb. or occasionally Petroleum. That is the way to group them. Always try to get a clear picture of the outstanding member of the group and then fill in the exceptions. As a start, the four remedies – Nux Vomica, Pulsatilla, China, Carbo Veg. – cover most cases of dyspepsia, but those that do not respond must be reconsidered.

GASTROENTERITIS

There are very few remedies to consider for acute diarrhoea and vomiting. For instance, for acute gastroenteritis poisoning, which is very violent and develops within a few hours, Arsenicum Alb., Carbo Veg. and Veratrum Alb. are the three to be considered. For more slowly developing diarrhoea and vomiting there are other useful remedies, a number of which are also described here. With a good knowledge of these remedies, most acute cases can be treated.

Arsenicum Album
In Arsenicum Alb. cases there will be very violent vomiting and diarrhoea, purging and vomiting at the same time. The patients say they get constant little gushes of diarrhoea which seldom stop, and which are associated with violent burning pains in the rectum. There is constant retching with a burning pain in the stomach, and extreme exhaustion.

These Arsenicum Alb. patients are at first extremely restless, and have violent distressing tenesmus after the bowels act. As the condition progresses they get more and more prostrated, they become very cold, look very anxious, and have marked tenderness all over the abdomen.

Between the vomiting, Arsenicum Alb. patients very often get relief from little sips of hot water, and the abdominal distress is relieved by hot external applications. In acute diarrhoea and vomiting they have a very dry mouth and may take sips of cold water, but this will be vomited at once, whereas a sip of warm water often seems to quieten the stomach temporarily.

During the acute diarrhoea, Arsenicum Alb. cannot lie still in bed, they get up and move about, and are liable to have an involuntary stool.

There is nothing very characteristic about the appearance of the stool, except that it is small, frequent, rather watery and very offensive.

Arsenicum Alb. is the typical food poisoning remedy. The attacks may be induced by any impure food, such as rancid meat, bad sausages, over-hung game or blown tinned meat. Occasionally an Arsenicum Alb. diarrhoea will be brought on by over-indulgence in ice cream in warm weather – from chilling the stomach when the patient is hot.

Carbo Vegetabilis

Patients needing Carbo Veg. do not have such severe vomiting as the Arsenicum Alb. patients, but there is a very violent, exhausting diarrhoea, with marked tenesmus and the passage of small stools, usually liquid, brown and offensive.

The patients have none of the restlessness of Arsenicum Alb. They look ill, the face is pinched, drawn and pale, and they are covered with cold, clammy sweat. They feel intensely cold, complain of the legs and feet being icy cold, and yet have a marked air hunger and cannot bear a close, stuffy room. They like to feel a movement of air.

There is burning in the abdomen, though not so marked as in Arsenicum Alb. and there is none of the Arsenicum Alb. dryness and thirst.

Another pointer to Carbo Veg. is that, in acute attacks, Carbo Veg. patients have a great deal of flatulent distension. They feel the abdomen is very distended, and pass large quantities of flatus. They have frequent eructations which give very marked relief. That is an important point as a distinction from Lycopodium, where in spite of eructating the patients still feel distended and there is no relief. It is important to remember that Carbo Veg. as well as Lycopodium may be needed in shellfish poisoning, although Lycopodium is the main antidote to oyster poisoning.

Carbo Veg. may be needed for patients suffering from food poisoning, or from eating too much ice cream when they are hot.

Veratrum Album

The third of these remedies is Veratrum Alb. Many cases requiring Veratrum Alb. have already had Arsenicum Alb. without benefit.

Arsenicum Alb. is considered the typical remedy for food poisoning with diarrhoea and vomiting, and is given automatically, whereas many of these cases need Veratrum Alb. and not Arsenicum Alb.

The indication for Veratrum Alb. is that there are gushes of large quantities of fluid material. There is as much vomiting and purging, or even more, in Veratrum Alb. as in Arsenicum Alb. The quantity of fluid lost is considerable. the stool is often odourless in Veratrum Alb.

The patients are always icy cold and bluish in colour. They are just about as pinched-looking as Carbo Veg. patients, and are drenched in sweat, in spite of losing so much fluid from the bowel. It is not quite so clammy as in Carbo Veg. but it is a cold sweat, and the patients themselves feel cold. The sweat is all over the body in Veratrum Alb., whereas in Carbo Veg. it is mostly on the face, hands and feet – not the general sweating as in Veratrum Alb.

Another indication for Veratrum Alb. is that after the bowels have acted, there is the most deathly faintness. In severe cases, with almost continuous vomiting and diarrhoea, the patients may become unconscious. In a patient with acute diarrhoea and vomiting, who is sweating profusely, with profuse discharge and a tendency to faint, Veratrum Alb. in a high potency should give rapid relief.

Camphor

There are one or two cases which present a less usual picture, and which will need other remedies. Occasionally a patient is seen in a late stage where the history seems to suggest Arsenicum Alb., but has progressed beyond the anxious restless stage to one of acute collapse. On enquiry it will be found that there have been alternating waves of heat and cold during the acute stage. In the state of collapse, the patient is icy cold to touch, although he complains of burning internally. He wants to be uncovered in spite of the external coldness, because of the burning heat internally. The skin is dry.

There is constant tenesmus, small dark stools, and the patient is on the point of collapse, pulse rate increasing, colour becoming greyish-blue.

These patients should respond very well to Camphor, given a high potency. They warm up very quickly, and when warm they can be covered up; while the surface of the body is cold they are much more comfortable uncovered.

Cuprum

Cuprum is another remedy that is sometimes useful in a case of diarrhoea and vomiting, with very profuse discharges from both the stomach and the bowel. The patients feel very chilly and have a mottled, dusky appearance, with blueness round the finger nails, and the extremities look rather dusky, but – unlike Camphor – with the chilliness, the patients want to be covered up. The skin is moist and there is a tendency to slight jerking of the muscles, jerking of an arm or jerking of a leg, and violent cramping abdominal pains. With the action of the bowels they are liable to get acute cramp in the gluteal muscles. They may get cramps in the calves of the legs and have a tendency to spasm of the hands, where the thumb flexes inside the fingers. These cases respond exceedingly well to Cuprum.

Lycopodium

Lycopodium is almost a specific for people who are oyster sensitive. In a case of violent diarrhoea and vomiting following a meal of oysters, Lycopodium is almost always indicated.

As a rule, Lycopodium patients have a great deal of eructation, which may be accompanied by vomiting. But they still feel uncomfortably distended in spite of the release of wind.

There is a great deal of rumbling and gurgling in the abdomen before the diarrhoea comes on, and then the most violent, liquid stool. These attacks seem to be more common in people who are habitually constipated, with a history that the attack has started with flatulence, distension, rumbling and a certain amount of colic. The first stools that were passed were rather lumpy and hard, and the later ones were liquid and accompanied by the passage of a large quantity of flatus.

Another symptom that helps in the selection of Lycopodium, in preference to any other remedy, is the fact that the abdominal distress is relieved by hot drinks. They must be really hot, not the warm fluid of the Arsenicum Alb. patients. A hot drink seems to get rid of a good deal of the flatulence and makes them more comfortable. As with Arsenicum Alb. patients, the abdominal discomfort is also relieved by hot applications

There is not the same degree of anxiety and restlessness as in Arsenicum Alb. Lycopodium patients tend to be anxious, but are much more miserable and depressed than the acutely apprehensive Arsenicum Alb. patients. It is much more on the history of the cause of the attack of diarrhoea than on the actual symptomatology that Lycopodium is prescribed.

Phosphoric Acid

The characteristic of Phosphoric Acid is that the patients have the most copious, watery diarrhoea, which is almost painless. It just gushes out and they may have complete incontinence. It is always very urgent, and the stool is almost entirely odourless.

The next indication for Phosphoric Acid is that patients seem unaffected by their diarrhoea. There is always a history of completely painless, watery diarrhoea, with extreme urgency and difficulty in controlling it. It may be accompanied by a certain amount of flatus, which is quite odourless. It may be induced after eating ice cream, or being chilled, or after a period of stress, and occasionally as an anticipatory diarrhoea from fear. Phosphoric Acid may also be indicated for patients suffering from diarrhoea after eating sour fruit. Patients requiring Phosphoric Acid rarely vomit.

Aconite

In conditions where Aconite is indicated, there is a history of a very sudden onset: the patients were in good health, then exposed to some food poisoning, or to being chilled or a similar situation which has precipitated the enteric attack. Occasionally an acute enteritis, which is the result of shock or fright in a highly nervous, excitable patient, will respond to Aconite; but the commonest cases are the result of chill or exposure. With their enteric attacks the patients suffer from acute burning and agonising, griping pain.

Aconite enteritis patients have an almost incessant urging to stool, with constant pain, heat and burning. They frequently have recurrent attacks of colic, with a burning pain in the rectum and acute tenesmus while the bowels are acting. As a rule there is a sense of relief in the bowels when they have acted, but the patients feel very exhausted and nauseated.

The stools in typical cases are always small and frequent, and consist mainly of blood and mucus. The blood is usually bright red, and the stools may consist of almost pure blood. It is a very acute inflammatory condition.

Always where Aconite is indicated, there is the extreme nervous anxiety and distress, a feeling of apprehension and restlessness that Aconite has in all its acute conditions. In acute bowel disturbances there is one symptom that is not so frequent in other Aconite conditions – the patients feel faint and may actually faint on sitting up. With the attacks of diarrhoea, Aconite patients are always intensely thirsty; their lips and mouth are dry and often have a slightly bitter taste. They may complain of a tingling sensation in the mouth. There is an apparent contradiction – with the diarrhoea they have intense thirst for cold water in fairly large quantities, but the colic is relieved by hot drinks, and the abdominal pain is relieved by hot applications. The abdomen is tender to touch because there is an intensely inflamed bowel, so any heavy hot water bottle will be resented, although warmth is comforting. Another thing about Aconite patients in their acute enteric attacks is that they are often pale and have a cold sweat about the head, but have a hot sweat when they are covered up.

A further distinctive symptom of Aconite is that, accompanying the enteritis attacks, patients have a certain amount of bladder irritation, but pass quite a large quantity of urine. The bladder is irritated but the urine is not suppressed. This is the opposite in Cantharis patients, for instance, who have scanty urine – a useful distinguishing point. One other symptom occurring with all Aconite acute inflammations, no matter where they are, is marked sleeplessness. The symptoms in most patients becoming suddenly very violently ill will be eliminated by Aconite, if given early enough. The symptoms are so intense that the highest potency can be used, and repeated frequently about every 15 minutes. If the symptoms are not subsiding within a couple of hours, do not continue with Aconite; some other remedy will be indicated. If the patient is responding, the mental anxiety subsides first, then the stools become less frequent and less painful. Continue the Aconite and the symptoms will probably clear in 18 hours.

Colocynth
Colocynth is indicated for a very similar sort of attack. There is a similar history of onset. It develops either from a digestive indiscretion or from exposure, and the symptom that always indicates the possibility of Colocynth is the intensity of the abdominal colic. This colic begins before the diarrhoea develops and is extremely severe. As a rule it starts as a somewhat indefinite griping pain, usually on the left side of the abdomen. Frequently before the diarrhoea develops, the colic tends to spread up into the epigastrium, producing intense nausea and often vomiting. This subsides a little and the colic spreads further down. There is then a violent, sudden urge to stool which is so urgent that the patient has the greatest difficulty in retaining the stool. When the bowels are acting, there is violent rectal tenesmus associated with generalised abdominal colic. One of the characteristic symptoms is that the patients often complain of a violent pain in the forehead during a stool, during this tenesmus and colic. As a rule they get relief from colic

after a stool, but it leaves a burning pain in the rectum and round the anus. That is the typical picture. Patients will occasionally get the violent urging to stool and feeling of inability to control the bowels unaccompanied by any colic at all, the colic developing only after the bowels have acted; but that is less common.

At first the stool is profuse and liquid, containing mucus which quickly becomes bloodstained, the mucus and blood increasing with the frequency of the stools. The next constant thing in Colocynth enteritis is that any food or drink tends to produce an attack of colic, followed by an action of the bowels.

There is a good deal of bladder irritation, with urging to urinate, and often a statement that while passing urine, abdominal colic tends to develop and then the urge to stool. Colocynth patients have acutely inflamed bowels, the abdomen is tender and they dislike any weight on the abdomen because of the inflammation; for that reason they lie with their legs drawn up, to take the tension off the abdomen. But they are more comfortable and the colic is relieved by hot applications and gentle, steady, firm pressure.

One outstanding difference between the Colocynth and Aconite is that there is not the same fear of death in the Colocynth patients. Colocynth dislike being disturbed, dislike being interfered with and would much rather be left alone. All Colocynth patients are thirsty, but that is so common in an acute enteritis that it is not of great importance.

One point, which is sometimes a help, is that with a Colocynth colic the patients frequently say that the colic is eased and made more comfortable by taking coffee or by smoking. Smoking tends to relieve the abdominal irritation in Cololcynth patients. This is exceptional and therefore of value. They are restless, which is a useful point, because patients requiring some of the other remedies are only comfortable when they are keeping still.

Given early, Colocynth should clear the symptoms altogether. If symptoms have been present for some days and the inflammatory condition in the bowel has been extensive, and the colic is tending to become less intense and the tenesmus greater, the remedy needed to follow will probably be one of the Mercury salts.

Mercurius
The best way to consider the Mercury salts is to take Merc. Sol. or Merc. Viv. as typical of them all, because in enteritis, considering Mercury or one of its salts is purely a question of intensity. Merc. Sol.

and Merc. Viv. are interchangeable, and one of these two is intended whenever the abbreviation Merc. is used. If the stool appears to consist of almost nothing but blood, the condition will respond better if the patient is given Merc. Cor. or Merc. Cy. If the stool consists mainly of mucus, there will probably be a better response from Merc. Sol. or Merc. Viv.

The main distinguishing point between Colocynth and Merc. Sol. is the fact that the colic has subsided or has not been present, and there is very much more inflammatory disturbance in the pelvis, colon and rectum, with the most violent, frequently recurring urging to stool. This is a Merc. Sol. characteristic. With this urging to stool there may be a feeling of nausea without actual vomiting, and the patients complaining that they feel intensely chilly. Merc. patients feel alternately hot and cold. There is severe rectal tenesmus before the bowels have acted. During the action of the bowels the tenesmus becomes even more marked and the action produces very small, very slimy, bloody stools, which feel as if they were scalding the anus. During the time the bowels are acting the patients feel even more chilly than before, yet often break out into a hot sweat on the head. After the bowels have acted, the tenesmus continues and there is no relief from the evacuation.

With their bowel disturbances Merc. Sol. patients have very little colour in their face. During the action of the bowel, they may become a little flushed with a hot head and tend to perspire, particularly on the head and face. They always give the impression of being toxic and their eyes are heavy. Their mouths tend to become unpleasantly offensive very rapidly in their attacks of acute enteritis, and the tongue gives the impression of being large, flabby, pale and shiny. During their attacks they complain of nausea with salivation, and that their saliva is unpleasantly sticky.

In most of these diarrhoeas the patients are thirsty for cold drinks, just as Merc. Sol. patients are in all their other conditions. The attacks of diarrrhoea are exhausting and the patients very quickly become weak and tremulous. With their recurring attacks of tenesmus they usually get urinary frequency, but not the same degree of bladder spasm and bladder irritability that occurs in some of the other remedies. If these patients have severe bladder tenesmus and rather scanty urine, Merc. Cor. or Cy. is usually indicated rather than Merc. Sol. If the urine is markedly bloodstained, Merc. Cy. is the remedy. With rather scanty urine, it is Merc. Cor. There is severe tenesmus in both.

Kali Bichromicum

A remedy which is not so often indicated in the acute stage, but which may be needed as a follow-up in some of these very intense cases, when the condition has improved a little but has not cleared, is Kali Bich. The main indications for Kali Bich. are cases having intense inflammatory disturbance in the bowel and very small, frequent stools with a great deal of blood, mixed up with a lot of mucus, where the intensity is subsiding, the tenesmus easing, the stool less bloodstained, and the mucus less watery and becoming thicker. Kali Bich. patients with enteritis have abdominal flatulence, not very marked colic, with considerable urging to stool. This is accompanied by straining and the passage of strings of mucus, very little blood; but after the passage of the mucus, intense burning in the anus and rectum.

Kali Bich. will often clear up that type of case. During this stage patients often feel very tired out and develop the Kali Bich. desire for stimulants. If the inflammatory condition has spread into the stomach and there is an acute gastritis with mucus, that is an additional indication for the administration of Kali Bich.

Aloes

In acute conditions the Aloes stools are typical dysenteric stools. There is a marked tendency for Aloes patients to develop incontinence. When Aloes is indicated, the diarrhoea is always associated with flatulence, and the patients have incontinence of the bowel when passing flatus or passing urine. There is a peculiar sensation experienced just before the bowels act. It is as if the whole pelvis had filled up, accompanied by griping pain in the abdomen. That may subside with the passage of just flatus without any stool, or else the patients think that they are going to pass flatus, and a little of the bloodstained mucus comes away almost unconsciously. Another symptom is a griping pain high up in the abdomen, spreading downwards with this feeling of filling up of the pelvis and intense tenesmus, as if the whole rectum was in a state of spasm. As a rule there is a sudden, violent evacuation of the bowels, with complete relief of the urging and colic by the evacuation. There is also a tendency to develop a prolapse of the rectum or very painful piles. Associated with the diarrohoea, whether piles have developed or not, the patients have a sense of heat and burning in the rectum. Their piles are relieved by cold applications and aggravated by greasy ointments such as petroleum jelly. Quite frequently Aloes patients will say that before the griping pain develops there is a feeling of disturbance in the abdomen, with gurgling in the bowel, tending to come on immediately after any food or drink, but particularly after food. In the acute stage, they say that any movement or effort to pass urine tends to bring on the diarrhoea, and they may have incontinence of stool with the passage of urine.

As far as general symptoms are concerned, Aloes patients are irritable with their abdominal conditions. They are sensitive to heat and complain of a burning sensation in the extremities, particularly their feet. They are usually thirsty in spite of the fact that fluids aggravate their diarrhoea. The tongue is usually clean and they may complain of a bitter taste. During the griping attacks the abdomen is tender to touch, and there is a good deal of general abdominal distension. In spite of the abdominal disturbance and aggravation after food, Aloes patients with diarrhoea usually have a good appetite, which is an unusual symptom. The diarrhoea tends to be worse in the morning, often quite early – 6 a.m. onward – similar to Sulphur. But in the Aloes patients the diarrhoea is attended by a feeling of fullness in the rectum and pelvis generally. They have more colicky pain than Sulphur patients and the urge to stool is more violent, accompanied by more flatus. As a rule, Aloes patients are more irritable than Sulphur patients. They have a peculiar state of dissatisfaction with what is being done for them, and a state of almost childish anger when the colic is developing. Sometimes this is a help in distinguishing between Aloes and Sulphur, as their heat and cold aggravations are almost identical. Sulphur patients as a rule like meat, and Aloes have an aversion to meat. Alcoholic patients occasionally suffer from a morning diarrhoea, which can usually be checked by having some beer before getting out of bed. This condition can nearly always be cleared up with Aloes.

Podophyllum
It is very difficult to distinguish Podophyllum from Aloes in the textbooks. At the start of the diarrhoea the symptoms of both are very much the same. Podophyllum patients have the same aggravation after eating or drinking, and the first sensation they have is the same kind of gurgling in the abdomen and throughout the bowel generally. They develop a similar griping pain after the gurgling has stopped, but it is much more colicky in character. They get a sudden urging to stool, which is much more acute than in Aloes patients. There is not the same tendency to develop piles, but there is a more marked tendency to rectal prolapse with the stool. Podophyllum patients experience a very violent, aching pain when the bowels are acting, which Aloes do not. This is a real distinction between the two.

In Podophyllum patients the stools tend to be much larger, much more fluid, and the flatus is mixed up with the fluid stool so that it is expelled noisily. The appearance of the stool may be anything from a watery mucus stool to a very offensive bloodstained stool. Practically all the diarrhoeas which respond to Podophyllum are offensive.

Aloes patients, as a rule, are more peaceful for a while after the bowels have acted. In Podophyllum, the colic continues for some time after the bowels have acted, with a feeling of exhaustion. The stool is very forcibly expelled. Often the patients feel cold, alternating rapidly with flushes of heat that spread over their backs. Another distinguishing point about Podophyllum patients with diarrhoea is that quite frequently, just before the bowels act, they are not quite sure whether they are going to have an action of the bowels or whether they are going to vomit. They may start retching and gagging, and then have a sudden violent, watery stool. Cramp in the thighs or legs may accompany the abdominal colic.

As far as the abdominal condition itself is concerned, there is very little to distinguish the two remedies. In both, the patients have abdominal tenderness and are not particularly aggravated by either heat or cold. As far as appearances are concerned, they are quite distinctive. Podophyllum patients with diarrhoea look ill, as if they were going to vomit, and they are cold, clammy and sweating. Immediately after an attack, they experience waves of heat, during which they may become flushed; but in the attacks they become cold, pinched and distressed.

They have a night aggravation, not early in the morning, as in Aloes. It may be any time during the night, but is usually about 3 to 5 in the morning. They get a definite aggravation from being bathed. Podophyllum patients are usually lacking in thirst and usually have a coated tongue, either white or yellow.

Cantharis

Cantharis is the next remedy that should be considered for very violent bowel inflammations. It is never needed except in the very acute stage. The stools are always small, frequent and burning, and consist of a mixture of mucus and blood with shreds of tissue. The symptoms felt by the patients before and during the action of the bowel are a very intense, abdominal colic and urging to stool, with general abdominal pinching pains. The colic continues right through the action of the bowels and is accompanied by intense burning pain in the anus and rectum. There is always intense straining, often with a degree of prolapse of the bowel. After the bowel action the colic subsides, but the rectal tenesmus and pains are often worse. During this period the patients often shudder with the pain, describing the sensation as if cold water was being poured over them, and yet inside they were being burned up. They get a good deal of bladder irritation, either frequent urging to urinate, or suppression of urine. There is always burning pain during the passage of urine, and often burning in the bladder after the urine has passed.

Cantharis patients are always anxious and restless. They are very pale, particularly during the pains, although they may become flushed in between.

If the inflammatory condition spreads up to the stomach, they are thirsty whereas, with diarrhoea, they are thirstless and have an aversion to all food or drink. The abdomen is usually somewhat distended and is always very tender to touch.

All Cantharis patients tend to have a general night aggravation. This aggravation starts in the evening and usually lasts throughout the whole night. The acute symptoms in these cases can be controlled with Cantharis but, as a rule, some other remedy will be needed to cure, and by far the commonest one to follow is Kali Bich. This is indicated when the colic is beginning to subside and the stools are beginning to get a little less bloodstained with more stringy mucus, but with the tenesmus persisting.

Capsicum

In the typical Capsicum diarrhoea, there is a history that the patient has a good deal of general abdominal flatulence. Then, before the diarrhoea starts, there is generalised abdominal colic, tending to become more intense while the bowels are acting. There is spasmodic tenesmus in the rectum, during the action, and after the bowels have acted this tenesmus becomes much worse. The first distinguishing Capsicum symptom is that with the tenesmus after the bowels have acted, the patient becomes intensely cold and thirsty for cold water. Yet if they drink cold water, it often produces a sensation as if they were almost frozen, with acute discomfort in the abdomen and general shivering. During this acute tenesmus they often complain of intense drawing pain in the back, coming on after stool. Nux Vomica patients experience a similar sensation before stool, continuing during the action of the bowels, but not after. The typical stool of Capsicum patients is a rather thin, very slimy, adherent stool containing mucus and streaked with very dark blood. The upper part of the large intestine is mostly affected, so the blood is dark in colour. The patients stress that the stool tends to be very difficult to clear away, as it is small, adherent and slimy. Associated with their attacks of diarrhoea, they complain of feeling very tired and sleepy, and they may be yawning and stretching during the interview. The lips are rather swollen, and dry and cracked, and the patients often complain of a sour, offensive taste. They are acutely sensitive to cold and sensitive to draughts of any kind, even of hot air. They are not usually thirsty, except after the bowels have acted, but drinking water produces the peculiar cold shuddering sensation. They are usually rather fat people and sluggish in their movements. They tend to be pale, but often become very flushed during the action of the bowels. One useful symptom is that in their attacks of diarrhoea they often develop a craving for coffee, yet, if they drink coffee during an attack, they become nauseated. If the diarrhoea persists, bladder irritation may develop. This is sometimes severe, though as a rule it is slight. Occasionally there is very marked irritation with constant straining, but retention of urine. This is not a suppresssion of urine, which distinguishes it from Apis and Cantharis, and which patients requiring either of these remedies may develop.

Nux Vomica
Nux Vomica patients may experience a feeling as if their back was breaking before and during the action of the bowels. The general abdominal symptoms in Nux Vomica patients are generalised abdominal soreness and colic. Before the bowels act, they develop a very intense rectal tenesmus, a constant feeling as if the bowels were going to act lasting for some considerable time before the action takes place. After they have cleared the rectum there is almost immediate relief. They complain of a good deal of burning in the anus after the bowels have acted. The typical stools are frequent, small and usually semi-solid, and are dark in colour, mixed with mucus and thin bloodstained liquid. The patients complain that the stools are hot, burning and offensive. During the attack there is some bladder irritability, but never difficulty in passing urine – just urinary frequency. The rectal tenesmus eases for a time after passing urine, but soon returns.

In their acute attacks, Nux Vomica patients always have very severe abdominal tenderness. It is always much more sensitive than would be expected from the degree of inflammation. They always have a thickly coated tongue, which may be white or brown, but is usually yellow. They complain of an unpleasant taste, usually bitter, but it may be very offensive, almost putrid. With their acute abdominal conditions there is always nausea to a greater or lesser degree, aggravated after food. A distinguishing symptom is that Nux Vomica are drowsy after meals, or sleepy during the greater part of the day, and then disturbed and restless at night. As a rule they are thirsty and very chilly. In their digestive upsets they are acutely sensitive to smell, also to jarring and motion, due to the abdominal tenderness. They are very irritable and become very sensitive to noise and often to light. In appearance, they are under-nourished. They are thin, worried-looking, very often sallow, and may be jaundiced.

CONSTIPATION

A common condition seen in general practice is chronic constipation. It may be due to irregular habits, often accompanied by over-use of aperients, leading to an inactive atonic condition of the rectum. The usual advice about habit and diet, including fruit, vegetables and bran should be given.

There are three homoeopathic remedies which may help. Where the patient rarely gets an urge to stool, and the condition appears to be one of insensitivity and inactivity of the rectum, Opium in the 6c potency will often correct the condition.

In patients who habitually take large doses of aperients, where there is an urge to stool but inability to expel it, there is often a good response to Nux Vomica 6c given three times a day.

Some patients have bouts of severe constipation which are associated with haemorrhoids, which are painful and bleed. Hydrastis in a 6c potency will usually help.

In each case the remedy should be taken three times a day until a good response is obtained, then reduced to twice, and finally to once a day as the condition improves.

HAEMORRHOIDS

The treatment of haemorrhoids depends on the local modalities. If they are inflamed and acutely painful, and the patients obtain relief from hot applications, then Kali Carb. is the remedy. If they are relieved by cold applications, Pulsatilla will usually ease the pain.

A certain number of patients complain of a continuous throbbing

pain in the haemorrhoids, which are hypersensitive. If they obtain relief
from cold applications, Lachesis is the remedy.

Chapter 7

Obstetrics and Some Gynaecological Conditions

From the obstetric point of view there are various remedies which are useful and which have clear indications. Where there is a delayed or prolonged labour there are certain remedies with definite indications, which give a very much easier confinement.

OBSTETRICS

Caulophyllum
Consider a confinement where progress is slow, the mother is having indefinite pains coming at long intervals, making very little progress, and is just becoming exhausted. If there are no individualising symptoms at all, a few doses of Caulophyllum 200c given at hourly intervals stimulates the uterine muscle and brings on a labour that has not been progressing. Caulophyllum will also bring on the labour peacefully and successfully for the patient who has some contractions during the day, which quieten down at night when she goes to sleep, with no further progress, and who is becoming more exhausted.

Gossypium
Gossypium is not a very well known remedy, but is very useful in a similar condition. There is a history of a mother who has had a certain amount of abdominal discomfort and a definite show. On examination, labour has started, but she is having singularly painless contractions. As well as being painless, the contractions are intermittent and accompanied by a feeling of intense weariness. Very little progress is being made and, again, there are few indications except that the pains are so tiresome and exhausting, and yet not acutely painful. The mother is getting tired out of all proportion to what she is suffering. That is the kind of case which responds to Gossypium.

These two remedies, Caulophyllum and Gossypium, are the routine remedies to give to stimulate the progress of a labour supposing there were no other indications to go on.

Pulsatilla

In slow labours the most commonly indicated remedy is Pulsatilla. The reason is that the Pulsatilla type of patient tends to get distressed during labour. They are very mild, tearful and apprehensive, their uterine contractions are poor and they become worried and anxious. They feel hot, become breathless and may feel faint, wanting the doors and windows open, or to be fanned, and they make very little progress in labour. One of the indications for Pulsatilla in these mothers is that with each uterine contraction they tend to have an increased feeling of distress and suffocation, and often palpitation. On palpating the uterus, quite a good contraction can be felt starting, the uterus hardening up, and then the patient experiences this faint fluttering feeling and the contraction fades. It is the emotional stress that interferes with the normal progress of the uterine contraction and prevents their making any progress.

Another confirmatory point is that, whereas in most confinements the mothers are intensely thirsty – they are working hard and their mouth tends to become dry and they are very thirsty – Pulsatilla mothers remain entirely or comparatively thirstless. That thirstlessness is a confirmatory Pulsatilla indication.

In that type of case Pulsatilla will soothe the patient. It removes the nervous apprehension and the tendency to faintness and palpitation, and it strengthens and regularises the uterine contractions. After making no progress for hours, given Pulsatilla, four doses a quarter of an hour apart, the mother makes steady progress and labour is completed easily.

Kali Carbonicum

The next most indicated remedy in that type of delayed labour is Kali Carb.

The Kali Carb. patient is a woman who is getting weary with the slow progress of her confinement. She is very tired and probably a bit chilly, and is liable to be irritable. The indication for Kali Carb. is the manner in which the pains develop. The contraction starts and then the patient develops a violent pain in the back, just in the lower lumbar region or at the junction of the lumbar region and the sacrum; it is a sensation as if the back would split open. As the uterine contraction increases, the pain, instead of spreading round the sides as described by a normal patient, tends to shoot down into the gluteal region and into the buttocks. With that extension down into the buttocks, the patient arches the back and is unable to make any voluntary pressure.

In their confinement all Kali Carb. patients tend to get general abdominal discomfort, particularly flatulence. If they can get rid of a quantity of wind – usually upwards – they feel very much easier and as if labour could progress, whereas until they do get rid of wind they feel as if they could not make any effort. After some Kali Carb., the patient loses the intense pain in the back altogether, the contractions become more regular and more forceful, and labour progresses satisfactorily.

Chamomilla
One of the chief indications for Chamomilla is the patients' inability to bear pain. Whether the cause be purely mental or an actual hyperaesthesia, they become distraught with the discomfort and pain that they are enduring. Their mental irritability seems to check the normal uterine rhythm completely. A pain starts normally, the uterus is beginning to contract and then, instead of it going on to a full contraction with the voluntary muscles coming into play, the patient shrieks out, 'I can't bear this any longer', and the contraction ceases. She cannot bear any touch or any kind of examination. Often a Chamomilla patient complains that the pains in the uterus radiate in all directions, very often down the thighs, which seems to annoy her even more, and she always feels that much more should be done for her than is being done. She is the kind of person who is always asking for hypnotics, or else forceps to end labour when the cervix is only about one finger dilated.

After a dose of Chamomilla the patient begins to have pains of which she is barely conscious. It seems to relieve the hyperaesthesia more than anything else. Instead of the pains driving her nearly distraught, she does not seem to feel them until the cervix is half dilated. It is not unusual to see Chamomilla patients in confinements who do not require any anaesthesia until the child's head is on the perineum, although in the early stages of labour the mother gives the impression that early sedation will be required.

Sulphur
Sulphur mothers are sometimes very difficult to distinguish from Pulsatilla mothers. It is an interesting point that a patient who has needed Pulsatilla during the earlier part of a confinement, if the

placenta is very slow to separate, will almost certainly require Sulphur and not Pulsatilla to bring it away.

The typical picture of Sulphur is that of a mother who is becoming very exhausted. She is very weary, and complains constantly of having distressing flushes of heat. It is not the same stifling, hot, faint feeling of the Pulsatilla mother. It is much more a general wave of heat, often associated with a feeling of intense coldness in the legs and feet. And, as a contrast to the Pulsatilla mother, although she is feeling so hot and sticky, she is very sensitive to any cold draughts, whereas the Pulsatilla mother wants the doors and windows open.

The next point about the Sulphur mother is that when the uterus contracts, she often complains of feeling faint. It is much more a sinking faintness, rather than the stifling, palpitating faintness of the Pulsatilla mother. Very often, accompanying the feeling of faintness, a commencing uterine contraction can be felt just fading out and the uterus becoming soft and flabby.

Another point that distinguishes her from the Pulsatilla mother is that the Sulphur mother is usually thirsty. One thing she definitely does not want is cold drinks – she wants something hot and stimulating and feels better for it.

Sepia
When dealing with the typical elderly primipara, with a rigid, fibrous cervix in a poorly developed, thin, weary and sallow patient, always consider the possibility of Sepia.

One of the distinguishing points about Sepia is that as labour commences, and as dilatation starts in the lower uterine segment, the mothers frequently complain of localised stitching pains in the lower part of the uterus with the contractions, and these stitching pains often stop quite a strong contraction from progressing. Sepia mothers often have a very acute, distressing backache with each pain. It feels exactly as if the back were going to break. They do not get radiating pains down into the hips, and this distinguishes them from Kali Carb.

As the pains become more severe, and are obviously just about as severe as she can bear, as the contraction reaches its maximum, the patient develops a weird shuddering, the contraction subsides and she lies back exhausted, cold and very often somewhat faint. It is more a feeling of weariness and tiredness than actually a faint. Before the shuddering sensation comes on she may complain of feeling too hot, and yet she wants to be covered up. The Sepia patient is one who cannot be allowed to get out of bed and walk about, particularly if the room is at all cold, because unless she is kept warm she makes no progress at all in her labour.

In these mothers, Sepia will help to shorten the labour.

Nux Vomica

There are one or two remedies which are not frequently required, but which have definite indications and are very useful when needed. One of these is Nux Vomica.

The odd symptom that distinguishes Nux Vomica is that every time the patient has a contraction, she feels that she must get out of bed and either have her bowels opened or pass urine, and makes no progress in labour.

This is an unusual symptom and is useful to remember.

Cocculus Indicus

There is another type of case which is difficult to treat, illustrated by the following. A patient was progressing in labour very slowly. She would have one strong contraction and then three or four of which she was very conscious but which did not reach their full potential. Then she would have another good contraction, followed by three or four more coming to nothing. She just went on like that for twelve hours, making no progress at all. In addition, she complained of a general congestive headache and a feeling of numbness in her legs, as if they were losing all sensation. The feeling of numbness is fairly common, but it was particularly marked in this patient. She was very tired and sleepy, and slept practically all the time between her pains. After receiving Cocculus, the patient became alert, the contractions regular and strong, and labour progressed normally.

Lobelia

Two other remedies should be mentioned, because they help a difficult type of case, the one with the failing heart.

A patient with a mitral stenosis, the highly coloured, florid patient who tends to become very cyanotic, with acute dyspnoea as the pains become more intense, responds very well to Lobelia. The cyanosis clears, the respiratory distress eases, and the tendency to acute oedema of the vulva, which is so often troublesome in these patients, is very much lessened.

Carbo Vegetabilis

The other drug for patients with a failing heart is Carbo Veg., and it is given on the general indications for Carbo Veg. The patient is tired out, the pulse rate is increasing, and volume poor. The contractions are becoming weaker. The skin surface is cold and clammy. There may be a history that there has been a tendency to oedema of the ankles in the later months of pregnancy, probably with very troublesome varicose veins, and varices of the vulva. There is blueness of the lips and a feeling of air hunger. The legs and feet are icy cold, and the patient wants to get warm, wants to be covered up all the time, but also wants to feel movement of air. In that type of case, where there was a possibility of a difficult delivery, the patient should have quite a normal delivery after some doses of Carbo Veg., which can be given in high potencies.

Phosphorus
One type of mother that causes anxiety is the Phosphorus patient, because Phosphorus are liable to postpartum haemorrhage. With any known Phosphorus patient it is advisable to give her Phosphorus before the child is born, particularly if she is showing any signs of distress towards the end of labour, to avoid the haemorrhage.

There is one odd symptom to remember. After the infant is born, and before the haemorrhage, the patient may complain of a feeling of acute emptiness in the abdomen, accompanied by intense heat running up the back and a certain amount of eructation of wind. In such a case give Phosphorus immediately.

POSTPARTUM HAEMORRHAGE

Prescribing for postpartum haemorrhage is very difficult. These cases are very acute and treatment is urgent, so it is necessary to know the remedies, and a good knowledge of the homoeopathic Materia Medica may save a patient's life.

Ipecacuanha
The most commonly indicated drug in a postpartum haemorrhage is Ipecac. The patients usually get a feeling of sudden, intense nausea and collapse. They look deathly pale, they feel extremely ill, even from the first gush of blood.

Sabina
The other drug that may be needed is Sabina, which has almost the

same symptoms as Ipecac., a sudden collapse and faintness, but without the acute nausea. There is just the same gush of bright red blood, although the Sabina patient has large blood clots and then gushes of blood alternating. The Ipecac. patient tends to get gushes of unclotted blood.

Postpartum haemorrhage is an urgent and alarming condition, but it very rarely occurs in patients who have been treated with homoeopathic remedies throughout their pregnancy and confinement.

ACCIDENTAL MISCARRIAGES

The commonest causes of accidental miscarriages are falls, jars or over-exertion, stresses or shocks. Working on these lines there are clear indications for homoeopathic remedies.

Arnica
Arnica is the remedy if there is a history of a fall, which has been followed by the commencement of either haemorrhage or uterine pain, but without any definite signs of an inevitable abortion – merely a threatening without a great deal of pain, but just a little oozing of blood or bloodstained mucus or serum. Alternatively, if there is a great deal of aching or pain in the uterine region without definite uterine contractions, but possibly with a slight sticky discharge, a few doses of Arnica given at that stage will almost always prevent an abortion taking place.

The 200c potency may be given, about half a dozen doses, four hours apart for twenty-four hours, and by next day the danger of abortion should have disappeared.

Cinnamon
Probably the next commonest mechanical cause for a miscarriage is over-lifting. Strangely enough, cases of abortion coming for that reason do not respond nearly so well to Arnica as might be expected.

The patients usually complain of a good deal of dragging pain – a feeling as if everything had settled down into the pelvis, and a good deal of tenderness in the region of the round ligaments, and possibly some blood loss. That kind of case responds very well to Cinnamon.

One distinguishing point is that the Cinnamon type of patient is usually restless. She is extremely uncomfortable; she finds it difficult to get a comfortable position and tosses about. Arnica patients are made very much worse by any movement.

Rhus Toxicodendron

The third common cause for an abortion is over-exertion, the patients getting tired out, being much too strenuous and finally having a threatened miscarriage. That type of case usually responds very well to Rhus Tox.

These patients have the general weariness and tiredness of Rhus Tox. They have general aches, particularly backache, very often in the part they are lying on, aches which make them restless and want to move. There is always a certain amount of anxiety, they are tired and nervous, and their pains are severe. It is the type of case where abortion seems almost inevitable; but if treated early enough with a few doses of Rhus Tox., all the symptoms subside.

These three are by far the commonest types.

Ignatia

Another case which presents in the accidental class is the miscarriage from shock – nervous, emotional shock – and it is necessary to differentiate between the effect the shock has on different patients.

With the acute emotional disturbance and acute hysterical reaction, the patients find it very difficult to keep still. They are either moving about, wringing their hands or weeping, and they start having irregular uterine pains. In that type of patient, the miscarriage is usually prevented by a few doses of Ignatia.

Opium

For patients in whom the shock has caused prostration, with dullness and depression, where they are completely overcome by it, the remedy is Opium rather than Ignatia.

Aconite

A third type is one where the patient suffers a terrible fright, and after falling asleep at night wakes up in terror. One such case was a woman who came downstairs and found one of her children standing in front of the fire with her frock alight. The woman was three and a half months pregnant. She dealt with the emergency, but that night she woke up in terror, screaming out, and within half an hour she had started definite uterine contractions and a discharge of blood. That is the kind of case that responds to a few doses of Aconite.

So far as these emotional disturbances are concerned, it is necessary to differentiate the kind of shock and the effect it is having on the patient.

IDIOPATHIC MISCARRIAGES

Sabina

Apart from accidental miscarriages there are women who seem to miscarry for no particular reason. A perfectly healthy young woman starts a normal pregnancy, and then miscarries about the third month. If there is no uterine displacement, and no reason can be discovered for it, there is one remedy that will often help and that is Sabina. The main indication is that so long as the patient keeps perfectly still there is very little loss, but any movement at all starts up a haemorrhage. That is the usual story in this type of miscarriage. The patients say that in previous pregnancies they stayed in bed from about the middle of the second month to the middle of the third month, and as long as they were lying still they were all right; if they got up and moved about again there was a little show. There is apparently no cause for the threatened miscarriage. The blood coming away is quite bright and fresh looking, and as a rule it has a normal tendency to clot. Usually, if the condition is progressing, the patients tend to get a good deal of dragging, forcing pain from a point situated behind the uterus, between the uterus and the lumbar spine, and coming right forward towards the pubis – the premonitary symptoms of a miscarriage. That type of case responds very well to Sabina.

These are the remedies that might be considered for routine work. Beyond that, it is a question of prescribing for each miscarriage as it occurs. For instance, in a patient with a low lying uterus, think of one of the remedies which has the sensation of the dragging in the pelvis, such as Sepia. If the patient is a hot-blooded individual, consider Lilium Tig. If the patient has albuminuria, think of one of the remedies with a relationship to kidney disturbance, either one of the snake remedies, or Terebinth, or a similar remedy. Where it is associated with an ovarian tumour, consider the supportive use of Apis. Otherwise, prescribing is purely on the local symptoms and any remedy in the Materia Medica may be required.

The constitutional medicine can be expected to prevent a miscarriage, provided there are no clear indications for any other remedy. For instance a Kali Carb. patient tends to miscarry very easily, and Kali Carb. should stop this tendency. They suffer from persistent backache, the uterus is low, and they are very liable to miscarry if they get over-tired.

The remedy that helps most women who tend to abort in the later months is Sepia, because they cannot carry the weight of the full uterus. It is lack of tone that frequently causes the seven-months miscarriage in that situation. Sepia is the remedy for the cold-blooded patient, and Lilium Tig. for the warm-blooded patient.

SEPTIC MISCARRIAGES

(*Note.* Such cases will be treated with antibiotics now. It is to the patient's advantage to use the correct homoeopathic remedy as well, since this will speed full recovery. Ed.)

The three remedies most frequently needed for septic miscarriages are Secale, Sulphur and Pyrogen, and the indications for them are very distinct. They all have a very offensive discharge and of the three, the one with the greatest quantity of discharge is Secale. It has a purulent discharge mixed with dark, decomposing blood. In Pyrogen and in Sulphur the discharge is less in quantity, less bloodstained, more purulent and more offensive.

Secale
Secale patients are very restless, very anxious, uncomfortably hot, and yet have a strange feeling of coldness in the abdomen. This is apt to be forgotten about Secale because it is looked upon as one of the hot drugs, and the fact that the patients complain of a feeling of coldness is confusing. They are always thirsty and they are very frightened. As a rule they have a dry skin.

Sulphur
The typical Sulphur patient feels very hot, but it is not a constant feeling of heat. They experience waves of heat with perspiration and very often feel cold and shivery up the back. Their sweat and everything about them is offensive. They are much more heavy and dull and toxic, and far less anxious and worried than Secale. They are usually thirsty, though the thirst is nothing like so marked as it is in Secale, and

they tend to develop a purple congested look of the lips and mucous membranes in general. They are often very restless and complain of generalised aching pain.

Both Secale and Sulphur patients are liable to get a high temperature and, in Sulphur particularly, the infection spreads early from the uterus out into the pelvic fascia.

Pyrogen

In Pyrogen cases there are more general toxic symptoms – increased general aching, headache, aching in the back, aching in the legs. The patients may develop an early pelvic thrombosis. They are hot and sweat profusely, but they do not experience the same waves of heat that are present in Sulphur.

Both Sulphur and Pyrogen may have rigors, but they are more common in Pyrogen.

LEUCORRHOEA

There are four remedies which are more commonly indicated for pelvic lesions than any others – Sepia, Sulphur, Pulsatilla and Sabina.

Sepia

With Sepia patients there is always uterine displacement, usually accompanied by a mild degree of pelvic infection, with a rather bulky, unhealthy uterus, usually in a multiparous woman with a relaxed pelvic floor. They may have a cystocoele or a rectocoele, and very often a torn perineum. There are two types of discharge, either of which may indicate Sepia. One is a thick, greenish, acrid discharge, usually a B. Coli infection, definitely purulent in character. The other is a much more milky, profuse discharge, the type associated with a chronic endocervicitis.

The symptom that indicates Sepia is the feeling of dragging down, bearing down, of weakness in the lower abdomen, a feeling as if the perineum or the abdominal wall must be supported. These patients are almost incapable of standing for any length of time because of the dragging, which produces a severe backache, so they are more comfortable moving about. The other Sepia characteristic in these gynaecological cases is the feeling of emptiness, often described as a kind of false hunger, with not much desire for food.

Sepia patients have a general visceroptosis and suffer from chronic constipation. Occasionally a case presents in which, with a marked retroversion of the uterus, there is a feeling of something pressing against the rectum and a desire for stool, often associated with very severe, troublesome haemorrhoids.

Characteristically Sepia patients are tired out, miserable and irritable. They get cross with their surroundings, they feel they are badly used, that life is too much for them, and they just cannot bear things. Their inability to bear things may either show itself as breaking down and weeping or getting very angry. They are chilly and very sensitive to any disturbance about them, such as sudden noises or anything similar.

Sulphur

Two types of case present indications for Sulphur. One is the patient who has had a mild pelvic infection, either an incomplete abortion, or a subinvolution of the uterus. The other has irregular periods associated with the menopause, with a mild degree of pelvic infection. In both cases there is the same sort of local discomfort. There is a consciousness of weight, fullness in the pelvis, the uterus is bulky, very often tender to touch – more often in the infected case than in the menopausal one.

Definite Sulphur indications are that the discharge may be yellow, yellowish-white, or even faintly bloodstained. But no matter what its colour, it is always a very unpleasant, sticky sort of discharge, and always offensive, and very often the Sulphur patients themselves are acutely conscious of this offensiveness. The discharge is always very irritating. It either produces a sensation of heat and burning or intense irritation, becoming very much worse whenever the patient is warm. One of the characteristics is that any attempt to bathe, although it relieves the patient temporarily, tends to increase the irritation later.

Another Sulphur indication is that with these pelvic disturbances the patients tend to have disturbances of the circulation. They have flushes of heat from exertion or stress, and very often after eating, quite frequently followed by shivering.

Pulsatilla

Pulsatilla is indicated in patients with a profuse yellowish discharge, not noticeably offensive, probably with redness and swelling of the vulva and an uncomfortable feeling of heat. The uterus is enlarged and the patients complain of a feeling of weight in the pelvis. There may be actual prolapse but, as a rule, there is only a slight dragging down of the uterus, often associated with a good deal of thickening along the broad ligaments and probably an enlarged Fallopian tube, which is surprisingly non-tender. There is always a feeling of unpleasant, often distressing, fullness in the abdomen. Sometimes it is very marked, amounting almost to a sensation of being bloated with great discomfort from anything tight around the abdomen. It is accompanied by a feeling of heat with a tendency to faint, particularly in any stuffy atmosphere. The patients are usually somewhat overweight. Occasionally the vaginal discharge is completely non-irritating, although that is unusual in a Pulsatilla patient. Most Pulsatilla discharges are quite bland, but the vaginal discharges are usually irritating although they do not get the intense itching of Sulphur.

That picture in rather a mild, gentle patient with the usual Pulsatilla likes and dislikes, its desire for company, dislike of being left alone, desire for sweet things, dislike of fat, gives indications for Pulsatilla. It will clear most cases without any local treatment at all.

These are only the key-notes of these remedies; they are to help to identify them easily.

Sabina

(*Note.* Antibiotics are the recognised modern treatment for venereal disease. Before they were discovered, homoeopathic remedies had proved very effective in such cases and remain a valuable supportive therapy. Ed.)

If a patient presented with acute gonorrhoea and cauliflower growths, most prescribers would give Thuja, and be very disappointed with the result. Thuja will clear up a chronic gonorrhoea but it does not clear the acute condition. The remedy for acute gonorrhoea is Sabina, and in Sabina there are two conditions. One, the frank gonorrhoea with a pouring greenish-yellow discharge, with masses of soft cauliflower growth all round the vulva and extending back round the anus. These cauliflower growths are, like most of the gonorrhoeal growths, soft and insensitive, which is the distinguishing point between Sabina and Thuja. Chronic gonorrhoeal warts are much smaller and more sensitive, and indicate Thuja. The Thuja discharge is nothing like so profuse, or so thick, and not so deep in colour; it is not the greenish-yellow colour, but pale yellow and more liquid.

That is the classical Sabina acute case. The other case with indications for Sabina is the patient with a uterine fibroid who has the kind of discharge associated with a fibroid – the sticky semi-purulent discharge. They are usually overweight, with a florid complexion. They become pale owing to loss of blood from the fibroid. They have profuse periods, followed by intermittent loss, and become steadily more anaemic. The loss gets less and finally stops, and they are clear for a month or two, with just a slight leucorrhoea. During that time they improve in general condition, their colour begins to return and then the haemorrhage starts again. That is the typical Sabina history.

UTERINE INFECTION

After these four remedies, there is another pathological condition needing another group of remedies. It is a mild uterine infection with a quantity of not very purulent but very persistent discharge. For this condition, with typical viscid, whitish or yellowish-white, sticky discharge associated with a mild infection of the cervix or the uterus, there are frequently indications for Hydrastis, one of the Kali salts, or Natrum salts. They all have a similar type of viscid, sticky discharge, and in all of them there may be a torn, eroded cervix, or just a mild pelvic infection with a slightly enlarged uterus.

Hydrastis
There are certain distinguishing points between the three groups of remedies. Hydrastis has that type of discharge, but it tends to have colour in the sticky discharge – it is deeper yellow than in either the Potassium salts or the Sodium salts. Also in Hydrastis the discharge is more irritating; there is itching and general soreness. In the case of an eroded cervix, on examination the cervix is very friable and bleeds very easily. It is this tendency to easy bleeding which is the indication for Hydrastis.

Kali Salts
The Kali salts have a similar type of discharge, but there are certain minor points that decide their individual selection. If there is a history of a sub-involution of the uterus and the discharge persisting since a pregnancy, the probability is that Kali Bich. is needed in preference to the other Kali salts. It must be remembered that in leucorrhoeas, the Kali Bich. discharge is more yellow than the rest of the Kali Bich. discharges. The nasal discharge, for instance, is rather like white of egg; this leucorrhoeal discharge is of much the same consistence, the same stickiness, but it is yellow.

Another point in favour of Kali Bich. is that with the bulky uterus there is a sensation of prolapse, a dragging down in the pelvis. The patients generally tend to be very much worse in hot weather, and in particular their dragging sensation.

The type of discharge in which Kali Carb. is indicated is associated with fibroids rather than with an infected uterus. It is much the same in character as the Kali Bich. discharge, but almost always the patient gives a history of excessive periods. Finally, all Kali Carb. patients have the typical Kali Carb. prostrating backache, a low-down sacral backache which feels exactly as if the back were going to break, tending to be particularly bad at a menstrual period. They cannot keep on their feet during the first two days of the period, partly because of the excessive loss but mainly because of the intense backache.

The indication for Kali Phos. in preference to the other Kali salts is the fact that, in addition to the typical discharge, Kali Phos. leucorrhoea is always very offensive. It is also excoriating, the vulva becomes quite raw. The discharge also tends to be more profuse in Kali Phos., and there is probably a secondary infection, possibly a B. Coli infection.

Natrum Salts

Of all the Natrum salts, the most frequently indicated is Natrum Mur., which has a very characteristic white-of-egg discharge. Apart from the ordinary Natrum general indications, the point that indicates Natrum Mur. in preference to the other remedies for sticky discharge is that it is intermittent. There are days when the discharge is profuse and very troublesome, and other days when there is very little discharge and the patient complains of acute dryness, burning, itching and smarting in the vagina.

Another characteristic of the Natrum salts is that with their leucorrhoea, as with their other discharges, they tend to get herpetic patches on the mucous membrane over which the discharge is flowing, either on the mucous membrane or on the skin surface. These herpetic patches burn and smart, and are seen on speculum examination of the vagina.

LEUCORRHOEA COMPLICATED BY MALIGNANCY

(*Note.* In any case where cancer is suspected it is necessary that the fullest investigation be carried out, and every form of treatment considered, in the best interests of the patient. But whether surgery, radiation or chemotherapy are used, homoeopathic treatment is always a valuable supportive therapy. Ed.)

Kreosote

The commonest remedy for the palliation of a malignant growth in the body of the uterus or in the cervix is Kreosote. The first characteristic is the typical malignant odour, easily recognisable; it is a most penetrating, indescribable sort of odour. It is present in all the remedies for malignancy, but is worst in Kreosote.

In Kreosote, the discharge is intensely irritating; the surfaces with which it comes in contact become almost raw, and they are extremely sensitive to touch. Always with Kreosote indications there is a purulent discharge mixed with streaks of blood, which is partly decomposed. There may be streaks of bright blood, but there will be black streaks in among it, and with this type of discharge, Kreosote will give great relief.

Carbo Animalis

There is another type with malignant ulceration of the cervix, where there is a much more watery type of discharge than occurs with malignancy of the body of the uterus. In Carbo Animalis the discharge is particularly irritating, much more extensively so than in Kreosote. The inflammation seems to spread down the thighs much more than it does in Kreosote. As with all malignant disease of the cervix, the discharge is bloodstained, but the cervix is not nearly so friable as in the typical Kreosote case. The discharge is very offensive, but not quite so penetratingly offensive as in Kreosote, and it seems to be more foetid than the horrible decomposition smell of the other. Then the patients requiring Kreosote have been fairly well-nourished originally, whereas Carbo Animalis patients have always been rather emaciated. On first looking at them they may suggest Sepia; they have the same sort of brownish discolouration of the face associated with Sepia, but Sepia does not help in malignant cases. In a patient with the Sepia exhaustion, weary, depressed and miserable, with the dragging down sensation, and the Sepia staining of the face, Carbo Animalis rather than Sepia will give greater relief.

Arsenicum Iodide

There is only one other remedy to mention and that is Arsenicum Iod. When dealing with a malignant uterus in a patient who gives the Arsenicum Alb. indications, extreme restlessness and anxiety, burning pains, incessant and excoriating scalding discharge, Arsenicum Iod. will give better results than Arsenicum Alb.

Chapter 8

Sleeplessness

There are no homoeopathic remedies which act specifically as hypnotics in the same way as those which are normally given for sleeplessness, yet they are very helpful when given on the right indications.

There are two remedies which may be indicated when the sleeplessness is caused by stress of apprehension, such as going into hospital before an operation, taking an examination, or before an important business meeting.

If the patient is restless, unable to stay in bed but must get up and walk about, or tries to sleep in a chair and then goes back to bed again, becoming exhausted and increasingly apprehensive, Arsenicum Alb. is the remedy.

If, with the restlessness, the patient is miserable and depressed, and afraid to be alone, possibly becoming weepy and slightly hysterical, Ignatia will help.

In other patients the sleeplessness is caused more by activity of their thoughts rather than fear. Patients in hospital will be worrying over their families as well as their own condition and its possible outcome. The examinees will be going over all possible questions they may have to face, and the businessmen cannot stop thinking of the next day's meeting. These patients will be helped by Coffea. They are acutely sensitive to noise. They become restless and may experience tingling sensations in various parts of the body.

Other patients, not unlike them, who also tend to become more mentally active and more sensitive to their surroundings in the late evening, and cannot sleep, require Nux Vomica. They become very irritated and angry by their inability to sleep.

Both Nux Vomica and Coffea are very helpful for the sleeplessness caused by excessive coffee drinking. (The coffee should also be stopped.)

Another type of patient similar to those requiring Nux Vomica is one who is oversensitive, particularly to pain. This person is helped by

Chamomilla. The main difference is the type of irritability. It is a much more petulant, peevish state rather than the angry irritation of Nux Vomica. Chamomilla is also helpful for patients who have been in the habit of taking sedatives, when it is desirable to bring them back to a normal pattern of sleep. They very often respond to Chamomilla during the difficult phase of withdrawal, when they are particularly irritable and peevish.

Opium is another remedy which may help those who are trying to leave off regular hypnotics and who are in a state of acute nervous excitability.

Sometimes, more particularly in children, homesickness may be a cause of sleeplessness. They feel the strangeness of their surroundings acutely and want to be with the family. They are really miserable, and in these circumstances Capsicum will help.

There are also patients who have had long periods of stress, or broken nights from looking after someone through a prolonged illness, and who reach the stage when they find it almost impossible to sleep. They will require Cocculus Indicus to help them back to a normal sleep pattern.

Sleeplessness is uncommon in children, but for the nervous, excited, frightened child who cannot sleep, Aconite is the remedy.

Belladonna is also useful for the excited child with a flushed face, hot head and widely dilated pupils, perhaps seeing faces or black shadows in the corners of the room after getting over-excited at a party.

Sleeplessness may also be caused by pain. In hospital practice, the homoeopathic remedies used for this type of sleeplessness are mostly determined by the nature and site of the operation, and are mainly prescribed for relief of pain rather than the sleeplessness itself.

After an abdominal operation involving the stomach, liver or gallbladder, the most useful remedy is Phosphorus.

The most commonly indicated remedy after appendicectomy is Rhus Tox., where the patient is restless. If the patient is flushed, hot, thirsty and wants to keep quite still, Bryonia is needed.

Sepia is the most useful remedy after operations on the uterus, and Apis after operations on the ovaries and Fallopian tubes.

Where there is post-operative distension of the bowel, Carbo Veg. is the most helpful remedy if the abdomen is generally distended, Raphanus if there are small, localised areas of distension.

In conditions where sphincter muscles have been stretched, such as cystoscopy or sigmoidoscopy, or after operation for haemorrhoidectomy, Staphisagria is the most frequently needed remedy, although occasionally it will not help and then Hypericum should be given.

Sometimes Nitric Acid is needed after haemorrhoid operations, when the patient is intensely irritable and complains of acute stabbing pain.

After breast amputation, if the patient complains of severe aching pain, Arnica will help, or if the patient is very restless, Rhus Tox.

For neuralgic pains, shooting, cramping pains, whatever the site of the operation, Mag. Phos. is the most helpful remedy.

For sleeplessness, the homoeopathic remedies act most satisfactorily if they are prescribed in low potencies 2 or 3 times a day, or 2 or 3 doses during the evening, with the last dose on getting into bed. They should be stopped as soon as there is a good response.

Arsenicum Alb. and Opium should never be given in potencies lower than a 6c. The other remedies mentioned may be given in 1x, 2x or 3x. The remedies that are prescribed for post-operative pain should be given in the 12c or 30c potency, commencing as soon as the patient has recovered from the anaesthetic, and the dose repeated every half hour to every 4 hours according to the severity of the pain, until relief is obtained.

When prescribing for sleeplessness from anticipation, it is not usually necessary to treat the patient for more than 24 hours before the event. This may be difficult to arrange for a patient who is in hospital awaiting an operation but, if it is possible, the homoeopathic remedy will give them great relief from their anxiety and distress.

Chapter 9

Pre- and Post-Operative Treatment

The use of homoeopathic remedies in post-operative treatment is determined to a very large extent by the type of operation.

EYES

Hypericum
The eye is an intensely sensitive organ, and patients are liable to get very acute pain. After an eye operation, Hypericum may be given for the relief of pain as a routine.

Aconite and Stramonium
If the patient has a marked nervous reaction, becoming very excitable, restless and distressed, as eye patients do, the routine treatment is to prescribe Aconite, when they will settle down quite quickly. The best plan is to give the Aconite frequently at 15-minute intervals in acute and very painful conditions.

If the condition is more acute still, after the first stage is over, the patient verging on delirium, the remedy that controls it is Stramonium.

These are the three drugs that help after most of the serious eye operations. Use the 200c potency in each case.

Coccus Cacti
After the removal of a foreign body from an eye, if the patient declares that something has been left behind, prescribe a few doses of Coccus Cacti. This removes the sensation of a foreign body, due to abrasion.

THROAT AND NOSE

Arnica and Symphytum
After any operation on the nasal septum, removal of turbinates or

submucous resection, the indications are almost always for Arnica or Symphytum.

Usually the patient will say it is exactly as if he has had a blow on the front of the face, which feels swollen, and that he feels he cannot breathe. These patients respond to Arnica. Occasionally a patient does not respond to Arnica, in which case use Symphytum.

After operations on the antrum, in the first instance it is wise to prescribe Arnica. Some of these patients suffer very severe pain after drainage of an antrum, and Arnica will give them almost immediate relief, although previously they were complaining that their face was feeling exactly as if it was going to burst and that they were getting pains right up the side of the face from the area that had been punctured.

Arnica and Rhus Tox.

For tonsil and adenoid operations the indications are either for Arnica or Rhus Tox. In Arnica, the patient wants to keep the throat as quiet as possible, and obtains relief from cold applications to the neck and cold drinks. As long as the patient makes no attempt to swallow, the throat is fairly comfortable. The Rhus Tox. patient has relief from hot applications to the neck and hot drinks to relieve the throat and, so long as he goes on taking little sips of hot water, the throat is fairly comfortable. He wants to keep the throat moving. If he keeps it still, it is very painful when he starts to move it again by swallowing. This is the ordinary Rhus Tox. aggravation from keeping still and pain on beginning to move again, and the ordinary Rhus temperature reactions – amelioration from heat as opposed to the Arnica amelioration from cold.

After 48 hours these tonsillectomies may have a very offensive exudate, dirty tongue and foul breath. Merc. Cor. will improve the condition rapidly in the majority of cases.

ABDOMEN – RIGHT UPPER QUADRANT

In the abdominal region, prescribing becomes a little more complicated, but there are certain broad indications to follow. In the majority of cases that have had an operation in the right upper quadrant of the abdomen there are indications for either Phosphorus or Arnica. Occasionally Carbo Veg. or Chelidonium are required for operations about the gallbladder or in the region of the duodenum.

Phosphorus

The indications for Phosphorus are a sensitive stomach, a tendency to bilious vomiting, pains in the right upper quadrant of the abdomen. The patients are thirsty with a desire for cold water. They have a certain amount of anxiety and fear, want company and dislike being alone. They complain of a burning pain in the affected region. That is the ordinary Phosphorus case.

Arnica

Arnica patients will probably complain that they feel as if they have been kicked under the ribs. They have a bruised pain in the affected area with very marked aggravation from any movement, and the breathing is shallow in order to keep as quiet as possible. They feel far too hot, and have very little thirst. If it is a gallbladder operation they have a tendency to become jaundiced. A few doses of Arnica will give them relief.

Carbo Vegetabilis

Carbo Veg. patients are obviously shocked and cold, with clammy skin. They very often complain of cold legs and feet, a feeling of extreme abdominal distension, the feeling being out of all proportion to the amount of flatulence. They have a choking sensation and like to feel a movement of air, and may ask to be fanned. There is not very much thirst, but they want their drinks hot. They have a feeling of extreme distension after any drink. A few doses of Carbo Veg. will relieve these symptoms.

Chelidonium

Chelidonium patients have much more acute pain in the right upper abdomen. It is stabbing in character, tending to go through to the back, aggravated by any movement. They are more comfortable with a fairly firm bandage round the affected area. They are thirsty, have a tendency to jaundice and a desire for hot drinks.

ABDOMEN – RIGHT LOWER QUADRANT

Rhus Toxicodendron, Arnica and Bryonia

Passing to the right lower quadrant – the appendix, ileo-caecal region, right iliac fossa – the two great standbys there are Rhus Tox. and Arnica for the immediate post-operative treatment. If Rhus Tox. is given immediately after the operation it will prevent much of the post-operative pain and restlessness. The differences between Rhus Tox. and Arnica are just the ordinary differences between these two remedies in general – Arnica with intense aggravation of pain, discomfort and distress from any movement, and relief from keeping still. The patients feel hot, too hot, and have a general bursting, aching feeling in the side. Rhus Tox. patients on the other hand are definitely restless and, although it hurts to move, they cannot keep still. They have a dry tongue, thirst, recurring spasms of pain, and a desire for hot applications, which give relief.

These are the routine remedies for the appendix region. One other very commonly indicated remedy is Bryonia, and it is sometimes difficult to distinguish between an Arnica and a Bryonia. In both cases there is marked aggravation from movement, the feeling of being too hot and the dislike of being turned over or touched. But in Bryonia the tongue is thickly coated, white and with a feeling of nausea, and there is always a constant thirst with a desire for cold drinks – that is the main differentiating point between Arnica and Bryonia.

Note. In the following discussion of serious septic conditions and intestinal stasis, it is certain that chemotherapy will be used. It is still in the best interests of the patient that homoeopathy is also used as supportive treatment. Ed.

Pyrogen, Crotalus Horridus and Rhus Toxicodendron

A different group of remedies is required to help an acute septic condition, such as a gangrenous appendix after surgery, and to talk about the complications of all surgical operations would cover the whole Materia Medica. As a routine, with no definite indications when dealing with a septic appendix, or even a fairly advanced peritonitis, there are certain remedies to consider. After a perforation of the appendix, with a sudden drop in temperature and increased pulse rate, the best prescription is several doses of Pyrogen, 15 minutes or half an hour apart. The results would probably be best if the Pyrogen is given before the abdomen is opened. If, when the abdomen is opened, there is a sloughing, haemorrhagic appendix which bleeds when it is handled and it is difficult to stop the bleeding, with a very offensive discharge, the best remedy is Crotalus Horr. Start this immediately after the operation.

There is only one other routine to give for these appendix cases. Where there has been a gangrenous appendix and next day there is a tendency to infection of the skin round the incision, this will very often clear up on some Rhus Tox.; it seems to have a strange affinity for that inflammatory reaction round such wounds. These remedies cover the majority of cases; the exceptional ones must be prescribed for on their individual symptoms.

INTESTINAL STASIS

There are several remedies to consider when dealing with a case of abdominal operation in which there are signs of stasis of the intestine.

Carbo Vegetabilis
The first and by far the commonest is Carbo Veg. There is the general Carbo Veg. picture but, in addition, the point that strongly indicates this remedy is that there are scattered areas of distension. There are loops of bowel which balloon out for a time and subside, and then it swells up in another place and subsides; it is not exactly a visible peristalsis, but rather an irregular distension in a Carbo Veg. patient.

Stannum
The next most common remedy for this condition is Stannum. The patients always feel deadly tired and exhausted. They have periods of complete quiescence when the abdomen is perfectly comfortable, although it remains distended. Then a slowly increasing abdominal discomfort begins, increasing to colicky pain that subsides suddenly. There is sudden relief and they are at peace again for a time. The symptoms indicating Stannum are the steadily increasing discomfort, and then the sudden relief of the pain.

Nux Vomica
Another type of case is one with acute colicky pains, first in one area of the abdomen and then another. Accompanying the attacks of pain are intense irritability, restlessness, a feeling of nausea, and usually vomiting – often a bitter, bilious vomit. Associated with these symptoms there is a certain amount of flatus being passed, and urging to stool, yet very little passing. These symptoms indicate Nux Vomica.

Opium
Patients who have generalised abdominal distension without colicky pain but with nausea, very often with vomiting, will be relieved by

Opium. The patient just feels nauseated and vomits a small quantity, which dribbles from the mouth. He is obviously very ill and no flatus is being passed at all. His appearance is congested, dark red or slightly cyanosed, not as in Carbo Veg.

Raphanus
This is one other remedy which is particularly useful in any case of resection of the bowel or a partial gastrectomy, in which there is a tendency either to an inactive stomach, or in which there is acute distension of the first or second part of the duodenum. There is an area of localised abdominal distension with colicky pain.

SPHINCTERS

Staphisagria
Another problem is the acutely painful after-effect of any interference with any of the circular fibres – any sphincters. If, after dilatation of any sphincter, there is residual pain, it is nearly always relieved by Staphisagria.

COLICS

Aconite
The only other conditions that can be treated as a routine are the colics – renal, gallstone and intestinal. They can be covered by three or four remedies.

The acute, typical colic, associated with agonising pain, often terror on the part of the patient, extreme restlessness, and a certainty that they are going to die, is relieved by Aconite.

Colocynth, Magnesia Phosphorica and Berberis
In addition, there are three remedies to consider – Colocynth, Mag. Phos. and Berberis. Colocynth and Mag. Phos. have similar indications. The patients feel as if the area is becoming increasingly constricted, with waves of pain coming to one definite painful spot, and a feeling as if the bowel is being twisted up almost to the state of bursting. Any movement aggravates the condition. They want to keep as still as possible, and obtain relief from both heat and pressure. In an intestinal colic, Colocynth is more likely to be indicated than Mag. Phos. Where

it is a renal or hepatic colic, Mag. Phos. is more likely to be indicated than Colocynth.

The distinguishing point of Berberis is again the typical colicky pain, but instead of the pain gradually increasing in one spot, it starts in one spot and tends to radiate either down the canal, or through to the back, or out in all directions from the painful area. It has much the same modalities, with aggravation from movement and relief from heat, but the patients are much more sensitive to pressure than Mag. Phos. or Colocynth, and the pain is aggravated by it.

Chapter 10

The Kali Salts

The six common Kali salts are Kali Bichromicum, Kali Bromatum, Kali Carbonicum, Kali Iodatum, Kali Phosphoricum and Kali Sulphuricum. There are certain points of similarity running through them all, but their differences are very definite. In trying to compare them, it is impossible to consider them all together; the only way is to take the remedies one after the other, take the outstanding characteristics of each one, and mention the similarities and differences of the others.

Kali Bichromicum

The Kali Bich. patient is a fair, fat, somewhat sluggish individual, either male or female. Their faces are rather puffy, and they give the impression of having an unhealthy skin; the majority have a tendency to acne. Their eyes are rather dull, they may have a yellow tinge of the conjunctivae and there may also be a blepharitis. Suppose the patient is a man. He will be above the average height and look strong and muscular. He is easily tired, and when he is tired he wants to stretch out relaxed in a chair and do nothing ; he is definitely sluggish and almost lazy.

Their complaints fall into three definite classes. The common Kali Bich. patient is the typical catarrhal dyspeptic. Others tend to get bronchitis and attacks of asthma. Then there is a third group of Kali Bich. patients who are not so fat or so heavy, who have more colour in their cheeks and have darker hair. These are the people who come along with fibrositis. There is one other condition in which Kali Bich. may be needed, but that person does not correspond in appearance to the typical Kali Bich., and that is the patient with migraine. A certain type of migraine will not respond to any other remedy but Kali Bich. All these types are now considered here in greater detail.

Among the general reactions there are apparent contradictions in temperature reactions. Most Kali Bich. patients tend to be worse in summer and to get fibrositis in hot weather. At the same time they get skin irritation and their acne tends to develop. The respiratory conditions, bronchitis and asthma, tend to be worse in spring and autumn. When they are actually ill, Kali Bich. patients often complain of being chilly and feeling the cold, and they are worse from damp cold weather and from being in the open air.

They have one or two time reactions during the 24 hours. In all the Kali salts the patients have an early morning aggravation; it varies in time but it is round about 2 a.m. to 5 a.m. In Kali Bich. patients it tends to be earlier, in Kali Carb., later. Kali Bich. patients feel worse on waking in the morning and their respiratory troubles are worse. That is not the early aggravation, but an aggravation at the ordinary time of waking. One other characteristic is worth remembering. Kali Bich. patients have an aggravation after food; they feel more uncomfortable, heavier and have less energy.

One other useful point is that they tend to have definite alternations of symptoms, their fibrositis will clear up and be followed by digestive troubles or diarrhoea, or migraine clearing up may be followed by eye trouble. Pains may move from joint to joint.

In typical catarrhal dyspeptics, the patients complain of catarrh tending to be very troublesome in cold and wet weather. With their colds, their noses and all their nasal sinuses get blocked up with stringy yellow mucus. The mucus may be white if the complaint is chronic. The more chronic it is, the more the mucus tends to be white; the more acute it is, the more the mucus tends to be yellow. There may be involvement of any of the accessory sinuses, but all have a typical Kali Bich. pain – it is a boring pain, as if a blunt plug was being forced into the affected area. The most common area to be involved with a pain of this character is the frontal sinus, and it is often accompanied by a severe general headache. There may be similar pains over the antra or just over the eyes, depending on which of the sinuses are involved.

In between the attacks the appearance of the throat is very characteristic. There is very marked deep congestion of the whole of the back of the throat, often with strings of mucus hanging down from the posterior nares, an oedematous appearance of the tonsils, uvula and soft palate. It is a very typical throat requiring Kali Bich.

The catarrhal condition may extend right down into the lungs, leading to capillary bronchitis with a very troublesome cough. One point that often indicates Kali Bich. is the patients' marked tendency to choke. With the bronchial irritation they choke on solids; they can swallow liquids, but solids make them cough and they may vomit. Expectoration is worse in the morning. They have a 2 a.m. to 5 a.m.

aggravation, but also get a later aggravation on waking at their usual time. In the morning they cough and bring up very abundant stringy muco-purulent sputum with difficulty. They often feel better out in the open air as far as the respiratory condition is concerned, provided the air is not too cold and damp. They say that the most comfortable thing is to get into bed and get as warm as possible.

They often complain of a sensation of coldness in the chest. This cold sensation is common to both Kali Bich. and Kali Carb. patients, but in Kali Bich. it tends to be precordial, and in Kali Carb. it is a general coldness throughout the chest. One of the commonest complaints with the respiratory condition is a pain in the chest going from the sternum right through to the back. Kali Carb. have stabbing pains in the chest, but not this peculiar pain that extends right through to the back.

If the catarrhal state spreads down to the stomach instead of the lungs, Kali Bich. patients develop a typical acute gastritis or gastric ulcer. They complain of loss of appetite and flatulence, with attacks of nausea and vomiting coming on quite suddenly. They have severe distension of the stomach with eructations and a very distressing sense of weight in the stomach after taking food.

Their food likes and dislikes are very marked. They have a very marked dislike of meat; they have a bad taste, and water tastes particularly unpleasant. Usually they develop a dislike of fats during their attacks. They often crave sour things and have a marked longing for beer. The chronic beer drinker is fairly typical of Kali Bich. In spite of their longing for it, it gives them a definite aggravation; it makes them sick and often sets up acute gastritis. They also have an aggravation from coffee. Practically all vomited material is sour; it is a very watery, yellow stringy vomit. Occasionally they vomit up a meal and, after the stomach is empty, start bringing up a quantity of glairy white mucus, but this is not as common as the yellow glairy material. In gastric ulcer, there may be blood. It may be fresh or stale blood, but gastric ulcer is not so common as acute gastritis. The patients tend to get hepatic congestion, a feeling of weight, and a feeling of heaviness in the right subcostal region associated with diarrhoea, with clay-coloured stools.

Kali Bich. patients are liable to develop a catarrh of the bladder with strings of yellowish white mucus in the urine. Where this condition is present, a strong indication for Kali Bich. is a peculiar pain in the region of the coccyx coming on during micturition.

The next type of Kali Bich. patient is the fibrositic. The most frequent cases in which Kali Bich. is indicated have acute fibrositic pains and they all tend to sweat. The leading indications are the wandering characteristics of the pains. One joint gets inflamed and tender, then it clears up and another starts. The patient is lying quite comfortably and suddenly gets an acute pain that does not last long. Although the pain occurs in summer it is better from heat and worse from cold; it is aggravated by motion and relieved by rest. Sciatica in Kali Bich. patients is definitely relieved by motion, though fibrositis is aggravated by it. The sciatica occurs in hot weather and is better from applied heat, but not to the same extent as the fibrositis. It is also better from flexing the leg, and is particularly sensitive to weather changes.

A certain number of patients suffer from migraine. The type calling for Kali Bich. has visual aura; the vision is blurred, dim or hazy. This comes on quite suddenly some time before the headache, usually clears before the pain develops, but may continue throughout the headache. These migraine headaches are one-sided, sometimes right, sometimes left, and the pain is particularly violent. Often it is situated in a small area in one or other temporal region. It is relieved by firm pressure over the small area. It is helped by warmth, and definitely better from hot applications. Often these headaches tend to recur periodically; they are aggravated by stooping or by any violent motion. Often they develop during the night and are particularly severe on waking in the morning. They are often accompanied by violent sickness in which the patient brings up the typical, white, stringy, glairy mucus in the vomit. That is the typical migraine headache, and it is quite different from the catarrhal headache which begins at the bridge of the nose, extends up into the head, is quite different in its onset, and is connected with the nasal catarrh.

Kali Bromatum

There are one or two conditions in which Kali Brom. is particularly useful. The majority of Kali salts tend to be fat, and Kali Brom. patients are usually fat and fair, lethargic, rather depressed, heavy looking and dull. In spite of this apparent dullness there is a certain amount of local restlessness. They have fidgety hands and feet and there may be a definite tendency to twitch. They often complain of being unusually sleepy, and that they fall asleep in their chair if they sit down; they are thoroughly drowsy and heavy. They often complain of a tendency for their hands, feet or legs to go numb, and often also of a sensation as though the legs are trembling. Associated with this and their dullness they get a fear of insanity.

Patients I always found very difficult to prescribe for, before I came across Kali Brom., were children who were not getting on well at school. They are dull and apparently lacking in intelligence, rather like Pulsatilla children, but they have too coarse a skin for Pulsatilla. The first indication for Kali Brom. is a tendency to develop acne. Severe acne in a child with no other definite indications will often clear up on Kali Brom. It is the same with acne during menstruation in a woman; if there are no other indications it will often respond to Kali Brom. Occasionally a girl of that type who gets very long periods should also respond to Kali Brom.

General Reactions in Kali Brom.

Kali Brom. patients are hot-blooded, worse from heat, worse in summer, worse in hot rooms. They are better in cold weather and, like all the other Kali salts, they tend to have an early morning aggravation, round about 2 a.m.

Associated with their unhealthy skin there are three pathological conditions in which Kali Brom. may be indicated. The first is when definite choreiform movements have developed after a shock or fright – an adolescent of that type usually responds to Kali Brom. The next, in advanced nephritis, the patient seems heavy and sleepy with a slightly besotted appearance and threatened convulsions, and Kali Brom. will often help. Then there is another associated condition in which Kali Brom. is useful; in a bad case of infantile diarrhoea, where the child is beginning to develop signs of meningeal irritation, and there is the very peculiar liquid diarrhoea associated with the meningeal symptoms.

Kali Brom. used to be prescribed in conventional medicine for controlling epilepsy, and a certain number of epileptic cases respond to it in homoeopathic doses. In women, there is a definite relationship between the period and the onset of the fits. They occur either during or near the period, and without that relationship I have never seen any good result from using Kali Brom. In both the male and female it seems that there tends to be an aggravation at the new moon. In all these epileptics requiring Kali Brom., both male and female, the fit is followed by a severe headache.

They have a curious aura before the attack, as if their whole body was swelling, whereas there is no actual swelling at all.

Kali Carbonicum

Kali Carb. is the most difficult of the Kali salts to grasp, with the possible exception of Kali Phosphoricum, but on the other hand, though these are the most difficult, they are also the most valuable.

The first impression of Kali Carb. is that the patients are soft. That is not the impression given in Kent – the Kali Carb. patient he describes is irritable, highly strung and nervous, but that is not the usual type occurring in the UK. They are not taut at all, but pale, soft, flabby people, easily tired out by any exertion. When tired, they always have backache, which compels them to lie down. They tend to be fat and often have flat feet.

Their mental picture is very much the same. The slightest effort of thought or excitement tires them, and they get into a peculiar state of mental confusion. They get up in the morning knowing they have a fair amount of work to do. They start something, and immediately think that there is something else they ought to be doing, so they leave the first job and dash off to do the second. They have no sooner started it than they leave it for a third, and so they get into a thorough muddle and end up by completing nothing at all. They also say that they are constantly misplacing things. For instance a man will explain that he can never find his notes in his office; he puts them away carefully enough but cannot remember where he put them. With that mental state they get the fear that they are going insane. They get hurried, make mistakes in their speech, miss words out, put wrong ones in, forget to finish their sentences, and so on. They become annoyed with themselves and get scared; they get annoyed with their circumstances, and become jealous and suspicious of those who are working with them. When they are in this state they are very difficult to get on with and often show a strange vindictiveness. Another constant complaint is that they get absolutely worn out with the slightest physical or mental effort. If they have any excitement they are quite exhausted and have to go to bed, and it takes them two or three days to get over it.

Kali Carb. patients have many fears: fear of insanity, fear of poverty, fear of the future and fear of death. Associated with this fear they get a very marked hoarding instinct. Kali Carb. patients are essentially possessive. They tend to hold on to everything; they hold on to life and are afraid of dying, even though their life may appear hardly worth living. They hold on to their husbands, even when they appear to dislike them; they hold on to their children, even when their children appear to be nothing but a worry to them, and when they treat them none too well. They hold on to their money and may be positively miserly, though this is often the result of their fear of poverty. Another thing that very often crops up, associated with this mental dullness, is the feeling of failure. They become timid and cannot stand up for themselves; if anyone accuses them of a mistake, especially a mistake they have not made, they simply lie down under it. This does not conform at all to Kent's picture of Kali Carb. Another important point about Kali Carb. patients is a very peculiar dislike of being touched; they simply cannot bear it.

Their usual complaint is a feeling that they are heading for a breakdown. They have a general catarrhal condition, they are susceptible to colds and usually have some digestive disturbance.

General Reactions in Kali Carb.
Kali Carb. patients are generally chilly, in fact they are about as cold as any remedy in the pharmacopoeia. They are not only sensitive to draughts but also to any cold air. Their complaints are very much aggravated by any exertion, mental or physical, and they are very susceptible to damp. An apparent contradiction to this aggravation from cold, and amelioration from warmth, is that they get an aggravation from warm drinks. What really happens is that they get warmed up by the hot drink and then, immediately after, they get chilled, and the aggravation is due to the subsequent chilling more than to the actual warm drink.They are usually more uncomfortable and more aggravated after meals.

These are the main points about them, except the typical Kali time aggravation from 2 to 4 a.m., and Kali Carb. patients have also the later morning time aggravation on waking. They always feel particularly unwell and lacking in energy when it is time to get up. Another point in Kali Carb. is the character of the pains. Wherever they have a pain it is the same type, whether in the arms, the back, the chest or the joints, and whether due to respiratory, digestive or fibrositic troubles. The pains are always very sharp and cutting, and are constantly flitting about from place to place. They are almost always relieved by heat, incredibly sensitive to cold, and mostly aggravated by pressure. Occasionally the pain comes on during rest and is slightly better if the patients move about, but if they move fast they are definitely made worse.

An old lady with a typical trigeminal neuralgia was about the best example of Kali Carb. I have ever seen. She was not only sensitive to draughts, but also so acutely conscious of any movement of air in the neighbourhood, that if a handkerchief was waved in front of her all the branches of her trigeminal nerve were mapped out in pain. The slightest movement of any sort brought on the pain, eating, talking, laughing, smiling, in fact any movement whatsoever. She was so sensitive to touch that she could not bear to wash her face, and she was the typical worn out, tired out, backachy middle-aged woman of the Kali

Carb. type. This is very like the description of Mag. Phos.; they both have the incredible sensitivity to cold, but the Mag. Phos. patient is relieved by pressure, whereas the Kali Carb. patient is aggravated by pressure. Mag. Phos. may relieve this type of neuralgia, but will never clear it up completely where there is this sensitivity to pressure.

Kali Carb. is as catarrhal as any remedy in the Materia Medica. The patients are always catching cold, and get a certain amount of nasal discharge when over-heated, either by exertion or by being in a hot room and going out and getting chilled afterwards. Kali Carb. also tend to develop a violent headache from the same cause. It is usually a temporal headache, either on one or both sides, and it is so acute that it gives rise to nausea.

The nasal catarrh tends to spread quickly down into the throat, and the patients have very typical dry, painful, hot tonsils with a large quantity of white, or sometimes yellow, tenacious mucus. There is early enlargement of the tonsillar glands, which are painful, tender and markedly sensitive to cold – this is a valuable diagnostic point. If this condition is not checked immediately, they tend to develop bronchitis, with a paroxysmal, dry, hacking cough. There is not much mucus, and what there is is mostly swallowed rather than expectorated. The cough is so violent that it is liable to go on to vomiting, and with it there is the typical Kali Carb. violent stabbing pain in the chest. There is also the usual 2 to 4 a.m. time aggravation.

Kali Carb. is hardly ever required at the early stage in pneumonia; it is after actual consolidation of the lung that it is needed. The indications are the time aggravation in the early morning, the character of the pain, the character of the sputum, the character of the cough, and the fact that the patients get definite relief from sitting, propped up and leaning foward. They have an aggravation from lying on the affected side, which as a rule is the right lower lobe. Associated with the pneumonia there is often marked dyspnoea, and they can only sip fluids, as they cannot hold their breath long enough to take a long drink. They cannot take anything solid, as it starts them coughing, and the cough goes on until they vomit. They always tend to get a peculiar pallid, slightly cyanotic, puffy look about the face. The great danger in Kali Carb. pneumonias is from a failing heart.

The remedy most likely to be confused with Kali Carb. is Hepar Sulph. Hepar Sulph. patients have the same respiratory trouble, the same type of cough, the same sensitiveness to cold air, the same involvement of glands, but do not have the same 2 to 4 a.m. time aggravation. This is much later – 7, 8 or 9 a.m., and they do not have the same puffy face. They are always much thinner, more drawn, more anxious-looking.

Kali Carb. patients always complain of a tendency to digestive difficulties, and the main complaint in every one of them is the tendency to flatulence; they get acute abdominal distension after food. They also have the very greatest difficulty in getting rid of this distension, which involves the whole abdomen, and is not merely a gastric one. They have a feeling of emptiness in the abdomen; they feel hungry and want something to eat, but are no better after eating.

Another quite frequent Kali Carb. symptom is a sensation of internal coldness in the abdomen, and, in respiratory troubles, a feeling of coldness in the chest. Often these patients strongly object to being examined because of being so acutely sensitive to cold, not only internal cold but external cold also.

Kali Carb. patients are liable to get colic. It may be intestinal, or it may be hepatic; often it is just a feeling of fullness and tenderness over the liver. They may have gallstone colic, but are more likely to develop cholecystitis than actual gallstones. Most Kali Carb. patients are constipated, and they frequently develop piles, which are incredibly painful, protruding as large masses and tending to thrombose. Occasionally they bleed, but the characteristic symptom is their extreme painfulness and acute hyperaesthesia – the patients cannot bear them to be touched.

Most Kali Carb. patients are definitely thirsty, and have a desire for sour things. In acute illnesses they have a desire for sweets. It may be for chocolates or sweets, or it may be an actual craving for sugar, which is quite a natural desire when over-tired, and such people are in a constant state of over-tiredness. As a rule there is an aversion to meat. Although it is not in the textbooks, most Kali Carb. tend to eat an excessive quantity of starchy foods.

They all tend to get dental trouble; they hardly ever come with a sound set of teeth. They usually have inflamed gums, an unhealthy, offensive mouth, and a rather suggestive pale flabby tongue. The usual Kali tongue, thickly coated at the root, may be present; more commonly they have a flabby, pale, swollen-looking tongue.

One other point constant to every Kali salt – and Kali Carb. has it more marked than any other with the exception of Kali Phos. – the patients are all aggravated after sexual intercourse; it leaves them absolutely exhausted. In Kali Carb. there tends to be an unusual degree of sexual excitement, and yet there is this absolute prostration afterwards. In Kali Phos. there is not the same degree of excitability, but the prostration is even worse.

There is very marked haemorrhagic tendency in Kali Carb. In the female, the periods may be too frequent and they are always very profuse. There is often a history of periods where the patient is never free from an oozing of blood, at times there is almost flooding, and then it eases down again into this state of oozing, but never really stops. The pathological condition is most likely to be a polyp or a fibroid.

It is repeated in all the textbooks that Kali Carb. is a dangerous remedy. Kent warns against its use in acute gout, but this is seen less often today, and the few cases I have seen have never called for Kali Carb. Many say it is dangerous to give it in a patient with enlarged joints, but that is simply not true, at least for rheumatoid arthritis. Many patients in whom there were definite indications for Kali Carb. received it in high potencies, and they did well on it. In pneumonia it has been given many times without dangerous results. It is, however, very dangerous in tuberculosis and the potency must be carefully chosen, as these patients do not stand the reaction well. In stomach conditions it has also been used many times without any bad result. Do not give Kali Carb. for gallstone colic in a patient whose constitutional remedy is Kali Carb. (The same is true in Lycopodium, where there will tend to be a marked aggravation if you give Lycopodium for a hepatic colic in a Lycopodium patient.) But if there are indications in gallstones for Kali Carb. in a patient whose constitutional remedy is something else, say Phosphorus, then Kali Carb. may be given.

If you have a Kali Carb. patient with colic, and no indication can be found for any other remedy, then give Kali Carb. in a very low potency. Aconite is very often indicated in a Kali Carb. patient with gallstone colic. This will relieve the symptoms, and when the pain has gone, it may then be followed up by Kali Carb.

(*Note.* Dr Borland also presented the following material on Kali Carb., which overlaps to some extent with the section above. However, it is not a direct repetition, and is included here because it contains valuable additional information. Ed.)

Kent states that Kali Carb. is difficult to assess. The impression I have of Kali Carb. patients is of pale, very chilly, fat, flabby, sweaty, slow people. They are very slack. They have slack joints, tend to have a fairly broad pelvis, and often have swollen ankles. Their ankles swell over their shoes and look puffy, more oedematous than fat. The next point – one links it up with their puffy, thick ankles – is the appearance of their face, which is pale and puffy. There is no colour, the skin is moist and gives the impression it will pit on pressure. They are heavy about the eyes, with swelling particu larly of the upper eyelid – not the puckered condition of Causticum. In colouring they are dark more commonly than fair. Another complaint found almost constantly in Kali Carb., no matter what else they are suffering from, is backache. It is similar to the Sepia backache, but lower down, more sacral. It comes on very easily from any exertion, walking or standing, and starts as an ache over the sacrum. Quite unlike Sepia, it tends to spread down over the buttocks on to the upper part of the thigh. It is relieved from lying down on a hard surface, and does not get the Sepia relief from sitting in a chair and pressure. Kali Carb. have to lie down flat before they get any comfort.

In personality, they are a queer mixture. An outstanding characteristic of typical patients is the fact that they are muddled. Their story is always one of confusion. They start to do one thing, leave it half done and start something else. They take on three or four jobs and finish none of them, and then become worried and agitated about it. If it is a man in business, he may start giving instructions to one of his staff, stop to begin dictating letters, then feels he must telephone an appointment. When he has started half a dozen things, and is getting on with none of them, he gets into a panic and nothing gets done at all. In that state, instead of slowing down and trying to get one thing finished, he becomes more agitated, more and more occupied, and never finishes anything. Another peculiarity about them is that they have a surprising inability to stand up for themselves. They get very irritable, but if they themselves are attacked, particularly if they are unjustly accused, they tend to become quite silent and cannot make any reply. They feel miserable and hurt, but they cannot fight back. That is the dull state of Kali Carb.

They are very apt to become jealous of anyone who is more capable, or who is helping them out of a difficulty, and they are often malicious in the statements they make about them. Another strange peculiarity, more commonly found in older Kali Carb. patients, is a strong hoarding tendency – they never throw anything away. It is different from the miserly tendency of some of the remedies, just an inability to part with anything. Occasionally the same sort of reaction will come out in another way. They become very possessive of members of the family, yet are unpleasant to them and make life difficult for them.

Another point is that they are acutely hypersensitive. They are very sensitive to noise, which irritates them intensely. When they are getting muddled they become annoyed about it. Even the dull patients are hypersensitive to noise, touch and always to pain. They are terrified of noise, which makes them start and they complain of a sick, sinking feeling in their stomachs. Afterwards they throb all over, even right down to their finger tips. The dull types of Kali Carb. will often say that they become much more muddled mentally after food, or even while they are eating, and will often yawn during a meal. They are depressed, sleepy and heavy, and are troubled by flatulence after eating. Practically all Kali Carb. patients have a fear of being alone.

They have an aggravation in the early hours of the morning of whatever is their particular complaint. If it is digestive, which is the commonest complaint in Kali Carb., they will be worse in the early morning, about 2 to 4 a.m. Occasionally a surprising symptom occurs in these dull patients. They dream of some of their friends, very often friends they have not seen for a number of years, and after the dream they hear of an illness or unpleasant happening affecting the person they have dreamt about. This has been confirmed many times.

So far as placing Kali Carb., they seem to come midway between Calcarea and Sepia. They have the same kind of mental dullness and chilliness as Calcarea, the weakness of the ankles, and the same tendency to sprain muscles from over-lifting, but Kali Carb. is almost certainly indicated for backache from strain. On the other hand, there are the family disturbances similar to those associated with Sepia, for example dislike of their family, but Sepia has not the same possessive tendency. They both get dragging in the lower part of the abdomen, and both get menstrual headaches, but in Sepia the patients usually have scanty periods, and in Kali Carb. excessive ones.

Kali Iodatum
There are certain constant features in all patients who need Kali Iod. They are hot-blooded, and definitely better in the open air. As far as appearances are concerned, both the chronic and the acute condition need to be considered.

Chronic Conditions in Kali Iod.
The typical Kali Iod. patients tend to be pale and delicate looking, with an unstable vasomotor system. They flush easily. They are usually fair skinned, and very often fair haired. The acute type are mostly more obese than expected: more flushed and deeper red than the chronic type, heavier featured, rather cyanotic and heavy lipped. Both acute

and chronic patients are depressed, very easily discouraged, and often having a definite disgust for life. They are bad tempered, irritable, and if annoyed tend to be abusive. They are restless, and if at all agitated this becomes more marked. If any attempt is made to control them they are very liable to burst into tears. If they are trying to make themselves understood, and feel incapable of putting thoughts into words, they get so agitated that in despair they burst into tears, because they are so worried about themselves.

There are definite times of aggravation in the 24 hours. They have the ordinary Kali aggravation early in the morning from 2 to 5 a.m., and Kali Iod. patients also tend to feel worse on waking up in the morning. They tend to waken with a headache, dry throat and general depression. They are susceptible to damp weather, and in spite of their general feeling of heat, and their aggravation from heat, they are upset by cold food, particularly cold milk. Another useful point is that they tend to get urticaria, and some also get asthma, both of which tend to be worse at the seaside. All Kali Iod. patients have an increase of appetite; they are hungry people, usually they are thirsty too, and they tend to get flatulence – all Kali salts do.

Kali Iod. is a very useful remedy in fibrositis, arthritis and also in sciatica, and there is one characteristic feature. If it is sciatica there is a point of tenderness over the sciatic nerve, with a diffuse area of tenderness much wider than the nerve. If it is arthritis there is the tender joint, but also a diffuse tenderness both above and below the joint. There is a definite heat aggravation both in the arthritis and in the sciatica; the patient wants the affected part uncovered, or wants cold applications. There is amelioration from movement, increasing the more that they continue the motion. It may be painful to begin with, but the pain steadily improves as they keep on moving. There tends to be a nightly aggravation. With the sciatica they are worse from lying on the affected side, worse sitting, worse standing, but better when moving about.

Acute Conditions in Kali Iod.
Kali Iod. is particularly useful in acute conditions of the eye and nose. Of all the inflammatory eye conditions, acute conjunctivitis of intense violence with blepharospasm is the most usual in these patients. They have the typical flushed face, marked oedema of the eyelids, all the outside of the eyelids is inflamed, the face round about is red, and the redness and swelling spreads up on to the forehead, so that it looks swollen and puffy too. There is intense photophobia, marked headache,

and the conjunctivae are red and oedematous. The discharge is thick and greenish-yellow, and on opening the eyes they simply pour tears. The patient complains of an intense burning pain, and often there is a very early tendency to ulceration of the cornea. This condition, when associated with aggravation from warmth and amelioration from cold, almost always clears up on Kali Iod.

Acute inflammation of the accessory nasal sinuses is another condition where Kali Iod. is frequently indicated. They are severe cases, with swelling of the forehead spreading down into the eyes. They have a peculiar deep red colour with intense bursting pain and intense fullness about the root of the nose, extending right into the skull. Associated with that is a very acrid watery coryza, with burning in the eyes and intense lacrimation, a tendency for the nose to become sore and raw and for the upper lip to become swollen. With these nasal conditions there may be small ulcers in the mouth, usually situated on the tip of the tongue. There is one confirmatory symptom – an intense pain at the base of the tongue when protruding the tongue. That picture always indicates Kali Iod. It does not matter whether the condition is conjunctivitis, frontal sinus, antrum or ethmoid disease; provided there is the heat aggravation it should clear up on Kali Iod.

For a hot-blooded patient with singing in the ears and no other indication, give Kali Iod. The same symptom in a cold-blooded patient is very often cleared by a dose of China.

Kali Phosphoricum
There is an important difference between Kali Phos. and the other Kali salts. In all the others there is a tendency to excess fat deposit, whereas most Kali Phos. patients are thin with a typical pale, waxy skin, usually dark haired, very rarely fair, and they are irritable and nervously and physically exhausted. They usually walk with a slight stoop, their movements are uncertain and there is a tendency to stagger. Sometimes this is due to giddiness, but more often it is due to actual weakness of their limbs.

Their mental state is one of great despondency. They are anxious, and almost always of the neuraesthenic type. In Kali Phos. patients the irritability is the irritability of weakness, exasperation, and a conscious inability to cope with their situation. In the state of irritability they usually break down, weep and become exhausted, and then develop tremor and fears, and feel that they will lose control and scream. They want someone to hold them, either to save their reason, or to help them to keep control of themselves. There are various other mental characteristics. They are always shy and nervous of meeting either friends or strangers, and are particularly nervous of going away from home. This is said to be home-sickness, but it is actually a fear of strange surroundings. They are not only shy of strangers, but suspicious of them. Another symptom quite frequently found in Kali Phos. and which has occurred in provers, is a fear of open spaces – a symptom that is often difficult to find in the Materia Medica. In spite of their nervous and physical weakness, Kali Phos. patients often become restless. They are also very easily startled and unusually sensitive to noise. Another characteristic is that, in spite of their apparent weakness, fear and exhaustion, a curious obstinacy characterises them. This is especially noticeable when advising them to take a course of action which will benefit their health. With their extreme lassitude and tiredness there is a definite dislike of life. They are depressed and yet they have a fear of death, and are never the type of people who commit suicide. This state often occurs after a long and severe illness or chronic debilitating disease when the patients have little resistance.

They are always pale and obviously ill, but under stress or excitement the face becomes flushed. They are also troubled with flushing after meals; with that they have a tendency to perspire, particularly about the head and face. Kali Phos. and Phosphorus patients all have a tendency to flush and get hot, and yet otherwise there are many differences between them. Associated with the weariness of Kali Phos. they have a peculiar pain centering at the seventh cervical vertebra, and involving the whole of the dorsal area of the spine. This is one of the most common complaints in Kali Phos. and occurs whenever they are tired. The characteristics of this pain in the back are that it is worse if the patients are lying down or sitting, and a little better if they move about gently, and it is associated with a general feeling of weakness in the back.

General Reactions in Kali Phos.
Kali Phos. patients are extra sensitive to cold, in fact most of their reactions are aggravations – they have very few ameliorations at all. Warm weather makes them worse, they are aggravated by food, they are usually worse in the morning on rising, always worse from real exertion, but occasionally slightly better from moving about gently; they are always hypersensitive to noise. As a rule, female Kali Phos. patients have a pre-menstrual aggravation, with definite relief when the period starts. They all have the ordinary Kali salts time aggravation in the early morning. They are particularly sensitive to touch, and any

emotional excitement leaves them trembling and completely exhausted, for instance any bad or startling news. They are aggravated by the stress of talking to people, especially to several people at once and yet have a fear of solitude. They have a fear of crowds, and in a crowd become tremulous and frightened. The main complaint is a feeling of general weakness. Associated with various pains and disturbances in their arms and legs, there may be definite nerve degeneration. Patients with multiple sclerosis may be markedly helped by Kali Phos. All these patients with numbness, tremor and pain are aggravated by exertion, but gentle movement seems to keep their circulation going and they feel better for it.

Practically all suffer from digestive disturbances, and there are certain characteristic points. There is a peculiar apparent contradiction so far as their appetite is concerned. Very often they have a curious feeling of hunger, more a feeling of emptiness, which disappears at once on taking food. They feel satiated immediately and as if the whole abdomen were distended. Even after a small meal – and Kali Phos. patients are never able to take much – they have bad flatulence. Yet, within a few minutes after eating, they again have the feeling of hunger. They are the characteristic nervous dyspeptics who are always nibbling. They practically all dislike bread, so most resort to sweet biscuits or to chocolates. They often waken about 5 a.m. with an acute gnawing hungry pain and eat a biscuit in order to relieve it. They suffer from flatulence which is very difficult to move, and which gives rise to colic. Some Kali Phos. patients have longer periods between the taking of food and beginning of discomfort. They suffer from definite hunger pains, but not as a rule from an actual duodenal ulcer; they do not have the immediate relief from food found in a typical duodenal ulcer. It is a nervous dyspepsia, not a true duodenal ulcer. With the digestive disturbances they have an unhealthy mouth, with inflamed and tender gums which tend to bleed easily, and they may develop a definite dental neuralgia. The tongue of Kali Phos. patients, particularly in their digestive troubles, is flabby and has a very suggestive mustard-coloured coating.

One of the likes and dislikes for food of Kali Phos. is often a craving for ice-cold water. This is a peculiarity, as they often complain of a feeling of coldness in the abdomen. Like all the Kali salts they have a great liking for sweet things, and like most Kali salts they also like sour things, and sometimes have a craving for vinegar. In a tired-out woman with backache, who likes vinegar, the first two remedies to consider prescribing are Sepia and Kali Phos. Both are chilly, both tired and excitable, both pale, both rather better for motion. In Kali Phos. the pain is mainly in the dorsal region of the back, in Sepia in the sacral region. Kali Phos. patients are rather worse lying down, while Sepia are better. Kali Phos. tend to be pale and often have rings which are nearly black round the eyes; Sepia are sallow with brown rings round the eyes. Like all the Kali salts, Kali Phos. have an aversion to bread and to meat.

Practically all these nervous, debilitated patients suffer from headaches, particularly those requiring Kali Phos. There is also another type of patient who develops headaches in which there are definite indications for Kali Phos., and that is the student who has been doing intensive study. The headache comes on during the night, is very acute on waking in the morning, often slightly better after getting up and moving about, and increases again in the evening. The headache is generally worse from cold, and greatly aggravated by noise. The pain is intense and seems to involve the whole head; the scalp and even the hair become tender to touch. Eating a little food eases the headache for a short time but it returns when the patient gets hungry. Wrapping up the head and keeping it warm gives relief, but any excitement or mental effort causes a severe aggravation.

Associated with the general tremulous weakness in Kali Phos. patients, they may have attacks of palpitation, with myocardial inefficiency and low blood pressure, and occasionally they have true anginal attacks. In these attacks, they complain that after the acute radiating pain has subsided, a sensation of numbness persists in the area of the pain.

Kali Phos. patients tend to present with recurring attacks of acute cystitis. In an elderly person, tired out and debilitated, and with a tendency to incontinence, Kali Phos. will often clear up the cystitis and re-establish the sphincter control. The patients complain of a burning pain during micturition, starting with the flow of urine and continuing after the flow is over, and the pain is usually situated in the bladder, not in the urethra. Considering the sugar-loving, tremulous, worn out, hungry, emaciated, debilitated patient, it is not surprising that Kali Phos. is frequently indicated in diabetic patients.

Female patients tend to have a scanty menstrual flow. If they have any leucorrhoea it tends to be excoriating and highly coloured. Quite frequently this occurs with a very acute ovarian pain. Two other points to mention are that, apart from the tendency to perspire on the face and head after meals or from excitement, the sweat glands are generally

rather inactive and these patients do not perspire easily. Also, their
sleep tends to be disturbed and they get violent dreams and nightmares.

Kali Sulphuricum

Kali Sulph. has similarities to both Sulphur and Pulsatilla. The typical
appearance is one of heaviness, weariness and sluggishness. The
patients are usually highly coloured and tend to have rather a coarse
skin. They are usually rather fat and slow in their movements. They
always complain of feeling tired, and the feeling of tiredness is often
due to laziness rather than physical exhaustion. They have a definite
aversion to work of any kind, either physical or mental, and are usually
depressed and sorry for themselves. They often lack confidence and
may be actually timid and, associated with their depression, complain
of a feeling of confusion and that their brains will not work very well.
In spite of their apparent timidity, Kali Sulph. patients are very often
impatient and liable to changeable moods – lively one moment and
depressed the next. They tend to become anxious about themselves,
think they are very ill, especially in the evening and during the night,
and take a gloomy view of life when waking up in the morning.
Encouraging them to a less serious view of their illness makes them
angry, and they are always obstinate. Associated with their mental
confusion they complain of giddiness and that their heads feel full and
their faces hot.

Another characteristic is their skin irritation; Kali Sulph. patients
are always troubled by itching – they itch practically all over the body,
eyes, nose, scalp and skin in general. They are also always catarrhal.
They tend to get catarrhal conjunctivitis; the eyelids are gummed up
and itchy, and there are yellow crusts on the margins. The discharge
also is yellow, as are all the body discharges, and they always tend to be
irritating and to itch, whether from eyes, nose, chest, throat or vagina.
There is an intense irritation of the nose and often some degree of
ulceration of the nose, which is aggravated in a hot room and in hot
weather. Kali Sulph. is one of the most frequently indicated drugs in
chronic otitis media, with the typical Kali Sulph. yellow irritating
discharge.

Kali Sulph. patients also tend to get haemorrhoids with the same
intense itching – perianal itching.

Warmth in general aggravates Kali Sulph. and they are always
better in the open air. They tend to be worse in the evening, and
definitely worse from exertion, as it makes them hot, and they perspire
and catch cold. They tend to stagnate when at rest, so they are better

when moving about gently. They are worse on waking in the morning, then they are sluggish and usually have a headache, and they are worse after food. One peculiarity, unexpected in such sluggish patients, is the intense aggravation that they have from noise. They tend to catch cold after a bath, whether it is hot or cold.

They are always liable to congestive headaches, with a feeling of intense heat and heaviness in the head. As a rule, the headaches start over the eyes and spread to the forehead. From there the pain spreads over the whole head, more marked on the right side. The modalities are practically the same as in Kali Phos. The headaches are bad on waking in the morning, worse in the evening, aggravated by warmth, worse after food, and worse during the menstrual period in women. The patients are sensitive to sudden movements or jarring, which aggravate the headache. They are better in the open air and from cold applications. Unlike most congestive headaches, they are better from pressure and better lying down.

Practically all Kali Sulph. patients are catarrhal, usually in the upper respiratory tract. When indicated, Kali Sulph. is one of the most useful remedies in respiratory catarrh. The typical cases in respiratory conditions look flushed and, with chest catarrh, have a very profuse secretion of mucus and râles all over the lungs. The cough is aggravated by eating and is eased by cold drinks and cold air, and the patient has a feeling of irritation low down in the trachea. The sputum is yellow and difficult to bring up. The state of the mouth is also typical, with yellow mucus on the fauces and a yellow coating on the tongue. They always complain of an unpleasant insipid taste, and especially complain of water tasting bad. In addition they may have the ordinary Kali Sulph. desires, the desire for sweet things, for sour things and for cold food.

Another condition in which Kali Sulph. may be required is arthritis, with general aggravation from heat, amelioration of pains from moving about and being in the fresh air. Associated is the dry skin, usually scaly in character and itching, and there may be an urticaria. The pains wander about, start in one joint, go to another and then go to a third. Associated with these pains, Kali Sulph. patients often complain of very cold hands and feet – this immediately excludes Sulphur, with which Kali Sulph. might easily be confused. Sulphur patients always have hot extremities, whereas Kali Sulph. have cold ones.

One other point is in connection with their sleep, particularly in febrile conditions, when Kali Sulph. patients have terrifying dreams of ghosts, death, robbers or murder, with violent struggling in their sleep. They wake up terrified. Sleep in Kali Sulph. is never restful. In some respects, Kali Sulph. and Rhus Tox. have similar symptoms, but Kali Sulph. are always worse for heat and Rhus. Tox. for cold.

Chapter 11

The Natrum Salts

Natrum Muriaticum

Not all Natrum Mur. patients fit the textbook description of having a pale, waxy skin. The majority tend to have an oily skin, not the waxy pallor which Kent stresses. They are much more likely to be people with a good colour in their cheeks, which increases during conversation or when they are embarrassed. Natrum Mur. patients are tense, they quickly become embarrassed, the pulse rate increases very quickly, and it is then that the skin becomes oily. They tend to develop small herpetic vesicles at the corners of their lips, along the margin of the hair and on the ears.

The textbook description of Natrum Mur. stresses the extreme emaciation, but it is the exception to see extreme emaciation. Natrum Mur. often have thin necks, but need not be thin otherwise. As far as colouring is concerned, they may be dark or fair. There is a yellow tinge of the skin, not very noticeable when they are flushed, but obvious when the flush recedes.

At a consultation, Natrum Mur. are often slightly embarrassed and self-conscious. They are apprehensive and yet they do not want to appear to be finding the consultation a strain. They have an appearance of self-assurance, almost of opposition. They are not the most friendly of patients and seem to be definitely on their guard. They will answer questions, usually fairly shortly, often abruptly, and do not give anything away at the beginning of the interview. After their confidence is gained they often pour out their troubles, but this defensive mechanism must be broken first.

Natrum Arsenicatum

Natrum Ars. are definitely pale and look slightly cyanotic, not sallow like Natrum Mur. They have blue rings round the eyes and the lips are pale. Instead of the herpetic eruptions that Natrum Mur. develop round the mouth, Natrum Ars. tend to get dry, cracked lips. They are much more nervous, much more frightened, but much less resentful than Natrum Mur. The nervousness of Natrum Ars. is revealed by their general physical restlessness. Their hands are restless, their fingers are restless, and often there is a slight twitch of their shoulder, arm or the muscles of their face during conversation. A certain amount of perspiration develops, but not the same greasy appearance of Natrum Mur. They are obviously tired. Observing these patients walking across the room, Natrum Mur. plant their feet firmly down on the floor, Natrum Ars. come in rather shyly and quietly.

Natrum Carbonicum

There is a general Natrum similarity with all patients needing a Natrum salt. The appearance of the typical Natrum Carb. patient, instead of the taut Natrum Mur., is much more fleshy. They are pale, with rather indefinite features. They tend to be more plump than Natrum Mur. and may be definitely fat. Natrum Mur. may be quite neat and trim, but Natrum Carb. will almost always have thick ankles. In conversation they tend to flush up, somewhat like Natrum Mur., but it is a much more blotchy redness.

The general impression given by Natrum Carb. is that they are less positive. They are tired, and waddle across the floor rather than stamp across it as Natrum Mur. do. While sitting in a chair they tend to slouch, whereas Natrum Mur. sit up and look people in the eye. One confirmatory symptom in Natrum Carb. is their reaction to sudden noise – it startles them and makes them acutely irritable.

Natrum Phosphoricum

Of all the Natrum salts, Natrum Phos. are the thinnest. They are generally underweight and often tall. The colour of Natrum Phos. is almost always pale, but they flush under stress, both cheeks becoming bright red.

The skin tends to be greasy, but not to such a degree as in Natrum Mur. Most Natrum Phos. patients tend to be over middle life, and are not so trim and tidy as would be expected from their general outlook and from the way they talk; they have rather lost their vitality. It is a great effort for them to remember details of their complaints. They are quite willing to help, but either cannot remember or cannot express themselves. Natrum Phos. are very hopeless about their condition. They do not think that much can be done for them, and usually come for consultation under some compulsion – someone has been urging them and they have had to come eventually.

Natrum Sulphuricum

Natrum Sulph. patients are definite characters. Practically all are fat and often rather under-sized. They usually have a high colour and may be florid, but with their high colour there is an underlying yellowness. In acute conditions they often develop a congested liver and may become jaundiced. They tend to get skin eruptions, similar to the Natrum Mur. eruptions, and they have a slightly greasy skin. The main impression that they give is of being rather miserable and discontented, and some are bad-tempered, although many just seem depressed and hopeless.

PERSONALITY

The main characteristic of all Natrum patients is that they are, without exception, hypersensitive. Take Natrum Mur. They are sensitive to noise, to surroundings, to music, to thunder and to people. That is constant throughout all the Natrum salts – there is a degree of lack of balance in them all, and in Natrum Mur. it may become extreme. They may either be over-conscientious, or may lose all interest in what they ought to be doing. They may either be over-affectionate or have no interest in people around them. They may either be full of fears – afraid of all sorts of things – or else they may get into the state when, they say, they are afraid of nothing. The same patient may change from one state to the other. One day he will tackle anything, the next day he will want someone to back him up in everything he does. One day he weeps from the slightest cause, next day nothing would make him weep. Natrum Mur. are said to have absolute intolerance of consolation; as a matter of fact they crave for consolation from the right people. They crave for understanding and appreciation, they dislike being touched, their pains are aggravated by touch.

They are always rather tense, and tend to be restless and fidgety. They move their feet, fidget with their bag, and complain that they are liable to get sudden muscular jerks. Comparing Natrum Mur. with Natrum Ars., Natrum Ars. are very much more nervous and have all sorts of fears, fear of disease, fear of impending evil, fear of something about to happen. Typical of the Natrum personality is that they are over-conscientious and complete what they have begun, though it is a great effort. If they undertake anything and meet with any opposition it makes them very angry, which exhausts them. Any mental effort is very trying for them. When occupied, they always have the feeling of

being hurried and working against time, which brings on a great sense
of mental and physical weariness. This is so marked that they will say
that after any mental effort they are compelled to go and lie down.
Becoming angry affects them so much that they tremble.

Natrum Carb. more nearly corresponds to Natrum Mur. than any
other Natrum salt, but the hypersensitiveness, particularly to noise,
music, thunder and people, is even more marked in Natrum Carb. than
in Natrum Mur. The reaction to any of these is either a reaction of
irritability, or else they have a severe attack of palpitation. The reaction
to music in Natrum Mur. and Natrum Carb. is sometimes rather
different. Music sometimes upsets Natrum Mur. emotionally; they
weep from it. The common Natrum Carb. reaction is the same.
Occasionally a Natrum Carb. patient cannot stand any loud noise, and
for this reason cannot stand a full orchestra, but they can tolerate quiet
music although they always get a certain amount of emotional disturbance from it. There is a degree of difference in their reaction to
sympathy and social relations. Natrum Mur. want to be looked up to
and thought well of. Natrum Carb. feel rather cut off from their
friends. They feel that their friends do not quite understand them, and
the feeling of being cut off often starts a dislike and criticism of friends
or relatives. Of the two, Natrum Carb. are much more sensitive to
people than Natrum Mur., and they take an unreasonable dislike to
certain people, particularly to strangers. Natrum Mur. on the other
hand are much more likely to develop a sudden passion for somebody.

The Natrum Phos. personality is one of being tired, discouraged and
rather hopeless, and a little discontented. That is their normal state; but
with interference Natrum Phos. become irritable and often very
impatient of advice, not of criticism as some of the Natrum salts are,
but of friendly advice. In spite of their weariness they often delay
seeking medical advice, and this is often due to a fear of illness. As a
rule they are rather restless and fidgety in spite of their weariness, and
they feel tense. Any mental effort, or effort of concentration, produces
this state of tension more than anything else. Natrum Phos. have the
critical side that is present in most Natrums, but it is much more liable
to be a criticism of somebody who is absent rather than the sudden
unpleasant reaction of the other Sodium salts to somebody who is
present. They usually have a grievance of some kind.

Natrum Sulph. patients are definitely depressed, and the depression
may go on to thoughts of suicide. During their depression they dislike
people; they do not want to talk to anybody or see them. They resent
questions and are suspicious of the questioner's motive. They may

appear sullen and yet, underneath this sullen exterior, they are apprehensive, fearful and anxious. Their discomfort and their apprehension appears to be more marked amongst people, and they are afraid of crowds. They often shun people even if they do not actually fear them. They often have a fear of evil. What form it is going to take they do not know; it is just a fear of something hostile to them.

TEMPERATURE REACTIONS

Temperature reactions are of definite help in distinguishing the Natrum salts. Natrum Mur. are typically hot-blooded. They are intolerant of heat in general, but are much more intolerant of any stuffiness than warmth; a stuffy room crowded with people really upsets them. They are also quite sensitive to cold and to draughts in spite of the general intolerance of heat. They are always better mentally out in the open air, but if they do any violent exercise and get heated up they perspire and the skin of the face becomes greasy, which upsets them.

By contrast, Natrum Ars. are sensitive to the cold. They like as much warmth as they can possibly get, yet if they have had an emotional upset, if they have lost their temper and are shaky, they are better in the open air. They are always worse in winter and are very sensitive to damp.

Damp cold upsets them intensely. They are aggravated by any exertion either mental or physical, and are usually definitely worse after food.

Natrum Mur. tend to get an aggravation of all symptoms round about mid-morning, 10.30 to 11.30 a.m., and they may get a sun aggravation, worse at noon and improving at sunset. Natrum Ars. have a definite aggravation on waking in the morning and another round about midnight.

Natrum Carb. are very much aggravated by cold, and very much better from heat, with one exception – they cannot stand hot sun on their head, it will always cause a headache. With that one exception, Natrum Carb. are worse from cold.

All the Natrum salts have thunder aggravation, but in Natrum Carb. it is more marked than any of the others. Natrum Carb. and Natrum Mur. have most marked times of aggravation, which are definite and typical. Natrum Carb. with gastric complaints tend to have an aggravation about 5 a.m. They often wake feeling very hungry, with definite gastric pain, and their only relief is to have something to eat. They are ameliorated by warmth but do not like great heat. They have a general aggravation at 5 p.m. Natrum Phos. are much more sensitive to draughts than any other Natrum patients. They are very sensitive to cold; they are miserable in winter and much aggravated by any change in weather. They are aggravated by damp weather or a damp atmosphere, and say that if they have a cold or a cough the symptoms are aggravated after having a bath. They get a good deal of digestive trouble too, and that is worse after a bath. They feel better after a meal. One other point is constant and very marked; they are always prostrated by sexual intercourse, and it is the only Natrum salt to have that symptom.

Natrum Sulph. are essentially hot-blooded, much aggravated in warm weather, and extremely sensitive to lack of air, a warm room, a stuffy room or a room full of people. They are very sensitive to damp, wet weather, and hot damp days exhaust them completely. In spite of their aggravation from heat, they are very susceptible to night air, particularly if there is a little mist about. Natrum Sulph. is a common chest and asthmatic remedy and people who get wheezy at night frequently need it. They have a tendency to an aggravation of most of their complaints in the spring due to the soft, damp weather. They are better when moving about and tend to be worse when keeping still. Natrum Sulph. tend to feel at their worst in the morning on waking. They are singularly irritable before breakfast, and feel better tempered after they have eaten.

They often say they feel better, brighter and more cheerful after they have had an action of the bowels.

FOOD REACTIONS

One outstanding factor in Natrum patients is their aggravation from milk. This is present in them all, in some more than in others. Natrum Carb. are the most sensitive to milk. All Natrums have an aggravation from rich foods, particularly fatty foods. Also an aggravation from starch, which is very much less marked in Natrum Carb. than in any of the others. Most Natrum Carb. are starch eaters, and they do not get the same degree of aggravation from it as the other Natrum patients do. In addition to these generalities that apply to all the Natrums, certain of them have aggravations peculiar to themselves. For instance, Natrum Ars. have an absolute intolerance for fruit; Natrum Mur. have not. Natrum Carb., Natrum Phos. and Natrum Sulph. all have an aggravation from fruit. This intolerance is most marked in Natrum Ars. and, after that, in Natrum Sulph.

There is a very marked aggravation in Natrum Phos. from sour things, and particularly acid things. They have the fruit aggravation, but only from acid fruit. A certain number of them have aggravation from alcohol, particularly Natrum Ars. and Natrum Phos.

Natrum Carb. have an aggravation from sweets, not found in the other Natrum salts. Natrum Sulph. have a very definite aggravation from vegetables, particularly green vegetables and potatoes.

Natrum Sulph. have an aggravation from coffee, which the others do not have. There is a good deal of apparent contradiction between their desires for food and their aggravations. In spite of all Natrum patients having an aggravation from bread, many of them like it. This is quite marked in Natrum Mur., less so in the others, but it is present in Natrum Carb. and Natrum Ars. Most of the Natrum patients have an aggravation from alcohol, more marked in some than in others, yet they all have a definite desire for beer and acid drinks. They all have an aggravation from milk, yet occasionally a Natrum Mur. patient will have a desire for it. They all have a desire for salt in varying degrees.

Sometimes there are apparently contradictory indications in the Materia Medica, which indicate a desire and an aversion for the same item of food in the same remedy. The desire and the aversion do not occur in the same patient, but in different patients requiring the same remedy. For instance, a Natrum Mur. patient may have a definite desire for sweets or a definite aversion to sweets. And again, some Natrum Mur. have a definite desire for meat, while the majority of them have an aversion to it. A certain number of Natrum Mur. have a craving for salt; others have an aversion to salt. If the patient has an aversion to salt, Natrum Mur. cannot be excluded.

Some Natrum Mur. have a real desire for wine or beer, yet some have a definite aversion to it. This is more marked for wine than for beer.

One peculiarity that is not recorded under many remedies, is that Natrum Mur. have a desire for soup. There are not many remedies that have a record of it, and Natrum Mur. is one.

Another constant feature of all Natrum patients is that they tend to be thirsty, especially for cold drinks, though a certain number of them have an aggravation from cold food. Natrum Ars. and Natrum Phos. have an aggravation from cold food, though they have a desire for it. Natrum Ars. have more desire for sweets than most of the others, with the exception of Natrum Carb. which also have this desire. Some Natrum Mur. have a moderate desire for sweets, but not any of the others.

Natrum Ars. patients often have a craving for bread, and almost always a desire for juicy fruits – an exception to the general Natrum reaction – and an aversion to fat. Natrum Carb. have similar desires to Natrum Mur., as well as a strong desire for sweets, and they have a desire for all sorts of stodgy, heavy, farinaceous foods. Usually they dislike coffee and have a very strong aversion to milk. Natrum Phos. often have a desire for eggs, which is not found in the other Natrum patients, and a desire for fish, particularly fried fish, and for all types of highly-seasoned food. The only exception sometimes found in Natrum Sulph. is that, in spite of their strong dislike for milk, they like boiled milk and often have a craving for ice cream. Natrum Mur. have a definite aversion to tobacco, but not so the other Natrum patients. The aversion to salt is more commonly met with in Natrum Mur. than in the other Natrums. The aversion to coffee is common to both Natrum Carb. and Natrum Mur. There is no record of it for the others.

DISCHARGES

The discharges of Natrum Mur. patients look very much like white of egg, and may come from any mucous surface. Natrum Mur. complain that the affected mucous membranes feel dry. With pharyngitis, on examination of the throat, there is discharge all over the back of the throat. But the patient feels it is dry, so that they have difficulty in speaking, and yet there is this sticky mucus all over. There is not the same complaint of dryness in the other Natrum patients with the exception of Natrum Ars., who complain of the same dryness. Other patients may have a burning sensation, but they do not complain of it being dry. The typical discharge of Natrum Ars. is usually rather watery, sticky and yellow, and it is practically always offensive. The offensiveness is not present in the discharges of Natrum Mur.

Quite commonly Natrum Carb. have an offensive discharge and so sometimes do Natrum Sulph. Natrum Ars. have the most offensive discharge. It is rather thin, sticky, yellow and offensive. Natrum Carb. have two types of discharge, one which is similar to that of Natrum Mur. It is white in colour, but not so thin; it tends to be lumpy and more ropey and stringy than the Natrum Mur. discharge. The other type of discharge in Natrum Carb. is rather thick, yellow and offensive.

In Natrum Phos. the discharge tends to be yellow, but is much more like pus than in any of the others. It varies between creamy colour and definite yellow, and the distinguishing feature is that it is an acrid excoriating discharge, and often has a peculiar sour smell. The discharges in Natrum Sulph. are usually thicker. They are yellowish-green, definitely purulent and usually fairly profuse. It does not matter which of the mucous membranes one is considering – eye, ear, nose, throat, rectum, vagina – the same type of discharge occurs in each of the individual patients.

TONGUE

The tongues in the five Natrum salts are fairly characteristic as a rule. Natrum Mur. tend to complain of the whole mouth feeling dry, and the tongue is either shiny and red, or else the shiny red surface is broken up by patches of white exudate. That is the typical Natrum Mur. 'mapped' tongue. In Natrum Ars. the tongue is rather flabby and toneless, with a quantity of viscid mucus in the mouth. The tongue resembles the typical Merc. tongue – large, flabby and pale, but without the typical ulcers in the Merc. mouth. In Natrum Carb. the tongue is very sensitive, slightly inflamed with a tendency to develop small blisters along the margins. It may be moderately coated, but it usually has a bright red tip, which is very sensitive to touch.

The Natrum Phos. patient has a thickly coated tongue, tending to be white or yellow at the root.

The Natrum Sulph. tongue tends to be very dirty. It is thickly coated, either dirty yellow or dirty brown. There is always a good deal of mucus and occasionally blisters, but the blisters are on the cheek or on the inside of the lips rather than on the tongue itself.

Natrum Mur. often complain of a salty taste, and Natrum Ars. of a bitter taste. Natrum Carb. complain much more of the burning sensitiveness of the mouth than of the actual taste, though if they have a definite stomach upset there is a degree of acidity. Natrum Phos. complain of sourness in the mouth, and Natrum Sulph. commonly complain of loss of taste and a feeling of disgust at the sliminess of their mouths.

DIGESTIVE TRACT

Natrum Mur. tend to have a sluggish digestion and high acidity, and complain of discomfort and a burning feeling in the stomach after meals. Associated with that, the majority of them suffer from obstinate constipation. Occasionally Natrum Mur. will be required for a patient with very chronic, persistent diarrhoea, particularly if they have a red, shiny tongue. But the typical Natrum Mur. patient is a constipated person. All the digestive disturbances in Natrum Mur. tend to be aggravated by eating. That is one of the points that distinguishes it from Natrum Carb. If they are suffering from an acid stomach they are very liable to become extremely thirsty. With the thirst they have a desire for cold drinks, which often relieve the stomach disturbances for a time. In abdominal disturbances there is a good deal of flatulence, and the patients are intolerant of any pressure on the abdomen. Both Natrum Mur. and Natrum Carb. tend to get a feeling of hunger. Natrum Mur. feel hungry between 11 a.m. and 12 noon, Natrum Carb. tend to waken feeling hungry about 5 a.m., and again have an empty feeling between 10 and 11 a.m. However, with a mid-morning hunger period the patients are more likely to need Natrum Carb. than Natrum Mur.

Natrum Ars. are much more liable to acute digestive upsets with burning pain in the stomach and vomiting, either an acute gastritis or a gastric ulcer. There is one peculiarity present in Natrum Ars. patients: they get a feeling of emptiness without a feeling of hunger, particularly in their stomach conditions. Associated with that, if they take any food, it immediately produces a sensation of nausea. With most of their gastric pain they develop thirst and want frequent small drinks. Even when the pain is not present they are hypersensitive to hot drinks, which always produce a burning sensation in the epigastrium. They have sour eructations and may have attacks of diarrhoea. These are usually fairly painful, accompanied by tenesmus. The attacks often start after the evening meal and may be precipitated by catching cold. The characteristic stool is bright yellow.

The outstanding characteristic of the Natrum Carb. digestive system is flatulence. All Natrum Carb. patients get a certain amount of flatulence and they all tend to have a lot of loud eructations. Also, very often, they suffer from troublesome waterbrash and heartburn. Most of the abdominal symptoms are relieved by eating. All Natrum Carb. tend to be hungry. They want food every two hours, and get a special hunger period about 5 a.m. and between 10 and 11 a.m. Another characteristic is their extreme susceptibility to milk. If they have an acute gastric upset and are put on a milk diet they will vomit, and if the diet is continued they will develop acute diarrhoea.

Most Natrum Carb. patients are thirsty and desire cold (but not iced) fluids. Apart from their acute attacks of diarrhoea they are constipated, but considering the type of food they like to eat, their flatulence and constipation are not surprising.

Natrum Phos. have one or two unusual symptoms. They get the Natrum sensation of hunger, but the circumstances are peculiar. They get a feeling of emptiness that is aggravated after meals and which is not relieved by eating. They also get this aggravation after a bowel motion. Apart from that, they get a sense of fullness after meals with eructations, which are definitely sour, more sour than any of the other Natrum salts.

There is a good deal of general bowel irritability in Natrum Phos. and a marked tendency to diarrhoea. The stool is usually greenish, watery diarrhoea accompanied by flatus. There is always marked urging before stool and a feeling of weakness in the rectum. There may be incontinence of stool.

Natrum Sulph. complain of fullness and weight under the right costal margin, as if the liver is heavy and congested, and as if it drags over the abdomen when the patients lie on the left side. Associated with that there is a good deal of nausea that develops after breakfast. It is not present first thing in the morning, but immediately they take food it develops, and with it they get the slimy feeling in the mouth.

Further down the digestive tract they get a tendency to a very congested, stagnant colon. They often complain of a feeling of weight in the region of the caecum and on examination there is a tender, full caecum. They have a slimy mouth and a tendency to jaundice.

Natrum Sulph. complain of frequent urging to stool. It feels as if they were going to have an action, but they only pass a quantity of flatus. Their aggravation time is 4 to 8 a.m. for abdominal conditions.

They tend to get morning diarrhoea and are not unlike Sulphur. It is useful to remember that in Sulphur diarrhoea comes on before the patient gets out of bed. In Natrum Sulph. the diarrhoea does not come on till after the patient gets up in the morning.

Another point is that Natrum Sulph. are very liable to develop piles, which are not very painful but which bleed profusely.

Chapter 12

Seventeen Important Remedies

Sulphur

The average Sulphur patient does not necessarily give the impression of the 'ragged philosopher'. Kent's description – and it is the same in Nash and Clark – is of an emaciated, scrawny, irritable, nervy, excitable patient. This type of patient is seen and does occasionally require Sulphur, but the more common type of Sulphur is a well-nourished person. They have usually rather more than the average amount of fat, a big figure, above the average height, and they give the impression of being very well satisfied with themselves. That self-satisfaction keys in with Kent's description and is, in fact, a lesser, slightly different form of it. They think their clothes are marvellous, and sometimes they think rags are beautiful. They are not very sure of themselves, yet they put up a good bluff and give the impression of being hale and hearty and self-confident; yet when cross-questioned their self-confidence goes. They are not really very sure of themselves and are resentful if found out. Then they are apt to become stubborn and rather obstinate, and to stick to what they have already said, even if it is not accurate. That tallies with the description in the books – 'taking up definite beliefs, and sticking to them'. Associated with that they tend to be untruthful. If a lie will serve their purpose they will lie without any hesitation, and sometimes it is difficult to decide whether they are deliberately lying or whether they are deceiving themselves. It appears that they can convince themselves of anything they want to believe, and they use that to serve their immediate purpose. These are all different shades of the typical Kent description.

As regards appearances, there is one thing pretty constant about Sulphur – one sees them very well turned out, often perfectly tidy, and often definitely proud of their appearance and not always without reason. This is a fairly common picture. In spite of this, they have always just missed being completely right, either their jacket does not sit well, or they have the wrong coloured tie, or their finger nails are dirty or something of the sort just gives the show away. Another constant characteristic is that they always have a high colour of the face and particularly of their mucous membranes. Their lips are red and they tend to have blepharitis and a mild congestion of the conjunctivae. That is the general appearance of individuals who may need Sulphur.

One thing constant in Sulphur is that they all have increased appetites. It is much more bulk than quality that they want. They enjoy their food irrespective of its taste, and tend to take large mouthfuls. They are definitely greedy.

A point which occasionally appears contradictory is the question of heat reactions. The Sulphur patient is aggravated by heat, there is no question about that. Yet some are apparently perfectly comfortable in a hot stuffy room with no air at all. In these conditions, they always look far too hot, their face is congested and sweaty, even if they do not complain of the room being hot. One thing they do dislike is a draught.

Calcarea Carbonica
The impression given by Calcarea is that they are soft. The outline of their faces is usually smooth. Very often in the adult Calcarea the patient is not overfat, and yet they give the impression of having a large head and a rather large face. Calcarea are always slow mentally and physically. They walk across the room in a very slow, deliberate manner. Another striking thing is the feel of their hand. It is a soft hand, very often slightly cold, not necessarily clammy, but it is boneless, soft and yielding, and they do not grip.

Then there is their slow mentality. They are slow in their speech, and pause to take in what is asked before they reply. They tend to get rather depressed. It is not an acute depression, rather a sort of condition where everything is in a minor key. If they talk about themselves, their difficulties or ailments, they are apt to weep. It is not a violent weeping, they just gently shed tears and are very sorry for themselves, and very hopeless.

They tend to go over and over their difficulties. Their friends complain that they are always referring to the same things, the same old difficulties, the same old worries, and they are always referring to them in the same old way. If it is the question of health, they repeat the fear that they are sure they are going to die, till the people who live with them become exasperated. It is this spinelessness that is noticeable. They have intense anxiety during the night, but this is due to a fear of the dark. They always have a feeling that they are mentally below the average. They are scared of things, and also have the fear that they are going to have a cerebral haemorrhage. This is a very common fear in Calcarea. They have particularly poor memories. They get confused and cannot remember the dates of their various illnesses, and they cannot remember any details of what they have read as soon as they put the book down.

Another fairly constant point is that they have quite a good appetite, though it is nothing like as good as might be expected from their appearance of fatness and flabbiness. They always have a good appetite for breakfast. If they miss breakfast, they develop a violent headache within 10 or 15 minutes, whereas if they have had some food they are quite all right. One other rather surprising characteristic, from their appearance, is that in spite of the fact that they are always complaining and making a nuisance of themselves, they are extremely sensitive. If they are told to pull themselves together and get on with things, they are very much upset by it. They are very sensitive to adverse criticism, also to any injustice or cruelty to others, which makes them go to pieces.

Calcarea people are always chilly and wear far too many clothes. If the room is hot, the skin is moist to the touch, yet their lower extremities are cold. It is said that Calcarea types have a fear of heart disease – it is wise to take this fear seriously as in many instances they are correct.

Graphites

This remedy has a very similar symptomatology to Calcarea, but there are differences to be noted in order to distinguish it. Graphites patients have rather large heads and faces, and tend to be fat, particularly about the face. Their features are heavy. Both remedy types tend to have rather pale mucous membranes. Their lips are pale and also their hands, but although a Calcarea occasionally has bluish extremities, Graphites is never blue.

Another difference is that Calcarea are definitely nervous when they come for consultation and have rather dilated pupils, which is not present in Graphites. Also in Graphites there is a droop about the eyelids as if they have been awake for several nights. It is a drooping and heaviness of the upper lids, not a narrowing of the eye.

Calcarea get tired out with any effort, particularly any mental work; Graphites get distressed, excited and worried. The Calcarea type gives up, whereas the Graphites type frets about it.

The typical Graphites patient finds it very difficult to make up his mind. He vacillates and hesitates over every decision. The Calcarea type usually sheds the whole thing and just does not bother. They both have a degree of depression. The depression in Calcarea is much more gentle and weeping than it is in Graphites. In the Graphites type there is a definite foreboding of trouble ahead.

Another thing that distinguishes the two is that Graphites tend to be fatter than Calcarea; patients needing Graphites are heavier in build throughout. The skin of the typical Graphites is not the very soft, moist skin of the typical Calcarea; it is much more rough, harsh and dry. In practically all their complaints the two remedies have a symptom which from the textbook is very alike – a feeling of a rush of blood to the head. In Graphites the sensation is a feeling of blood flowing up from the feet, as if the head would burst, and there is often epistaxis. In Calcarea it starts in the abdomen and, from there, surges up into the neck, not so much into the head as in Graphites.

Another distinguishing point is that Graphites have a peculiar sensitiveness to music, not present in Calcarea. Calcarea are often musical, but they do not have that same liability to weep when listening to music which is noticeable in Graphites. A further point to look for in Graphites, either at a consultation or in their history, is a skin disease with a honey-like discharge, yellow, slightly sticky, and most commonly found at the back of the ears, round the side of the nose or at the back of the neck round the hair. Another point that sometimes distinguishes Graphites from Calcarea is that many of these Graphites patients are singularly critical. Calcarea, provided they have had a good breakfast, are alert in the mornings. Graphites are slow and dull in the mornings, and tend to wake up in the evenings. This is a definite contrast.

In both of these remedies the patients tend to be constipated. Calcarea usually feel at their best while constipated; they do not get headaches or feel heavy. Graphites are disturbed by constipation; they feel uncomfortable, and are better when their bowels are acting regularly.

Thuja

Without exception, the Thuja patients I have seen have been fair-haired and with a fine skin, very much the sort of appearance seen in a pre-tuberculosis patient, fair fine hair, fine skin and rather delicate, with variable colour.

The classical description of Thuja is one of intense irritability and bad temper, depression and a definite loathing of life. That is not the Thuja familiar to me. Thuja patients are singularly well mannered;

they are sensitive, polite and grateful. They do get depressed, the depression usually arising from a consciousness that they are not doing everything that they ought to be doing, or they are not progressing as fast as they ought to be with the attention they are getting; or else they feel they are a trouble to their relatives because they require attention.

They are definitely impatient people. They like things done fairly fast and get impatient with those who are slow. In the Thuja patients I have seen there has always been a tendency to muddled thinking. When talking to them they are very polite, and want to do all they can to help. They hunt for the exact word to tell their symptoms. If they cannot find the exact word at first, they come back to it later and say that is the word they wanted. When writing letters they often complain that they miss words out or misspell them, and it worries them. This may become more marked and they begin to leave things undone. An even more marked symptom in children is that they stop in the middle of something because their attention wanders, and they have to be constantly reminded to go on with what they are doing.

A fairly constant symptom is that, in spite of being affectionate, they have a definite dislike of any contact with strangers. They often shrink when anyone comes near, and do not want to be touched. This is accentuated if there is any mental breakdown; they feel brittle, but even in the normal state they have this dislike of people touching them. They are very individualistic, but are not likely to make a mark in the world, and they do not like to have their privacy imposed upon.

All Thuja patients are truthful and scrupulous in everything they do. They are conscientious in the way they carry out anything they undertake, even to the last detail, unless their attention wanders. If it does and they omit something, they get very upset about it. They are very sensitive and they also become angry. Ordinarily big things which anyone would be justified in being angry about do not aggravate them, yet some quite minor thing makes them strangely angry. That is my impression of the typical Thuja patient.

Psorinum

Practically all Psorinum patients feel at their best immediately before they are going to be ill – one of the best key-notes for this remedy. Suppose they have a racking headache: they say that the day before they felt exceptionally well and so knew that they were going to have a headache. This is similarly true if they are going to have a cold or any other illness.

The appearance is characteristic. They are usually thin or on the thin side. They always have a very harsh, dry, cold skin, which gives the impression of being dirty. They are particularly susceptible to cold east winds or working in water. The skin cracks and peels, with deep fissures in the fingers and small cracks across the cheeks, which may actually bleed. They always tend to have very sensitive eyes that get red and inflamed in any irritant atmosphere, dust, wind or smoke. They often have a history of recurring styes and chronic blepharitis.

Causticum

Two other remedies, almost as similar as Calcarea and Graphites, are Causticum and Phosphorus. Yet from the point of view of prescribing, they are very different. The best way of considering them is to take their points of similarity first, and then to take up their differences.

Patients who may need either Causticum or Phosphorus have one thing in common: they are liable to develop colds and to lose their voice. Both have a twilight aggravation; they tend to get nervous and apprehensive in the evening just when the light is beginning to fail. Both have a tendency to tremble and also a tendency to stiffness, particularly when they start to move. These are the most common points.

There are certain other similarities. Consider Causticum first.

Typical Causticum patients have rather fine delicate features and extremities, and are usually pale. It is that pallor that gives the first distinguishing point. It is a peculiar greyish pallor, rather like the kind of greyness seen if a piece of porcelain breaks and this greyness is under the porcelain glaze. Another indication is a certain amount of pigmentation over the temples, a yellowish tinge. Often there are small warty growths near the eyes. These are the visible indications for Causticum.

They are definitely anxious individuals, particularly about their friends. For instance, if friends are late they get worried about them in case something has happened to them. They are also rather shy and timid. They try to conceal their anxiety, either about their affairs or their health, by a slightly nervous laugh. Their memory is weak. They find difficulty in telling their story, and the effort of concentration produces a very unpleasant feeling of tension in their heads. They frequently have disturbed nights, with a general feeling of restlessness and discomfort. Their eyes look heavy. The lids are usually thin and wrinkled; they are not puffy at all and yet there is a definite droop about them and there may be an actual ptosis.

Causticum give the impression of being thin, but it is much more a thinness of the face and neck than of the extremities, and most of them have peculiarly flabby, toneless abdominal muscles. They are definitely irritable people, and often slightly difficult to deal with. They have a fairly good opinion of themselves – if their wishes are not carried out accurately and rapidly they are apt to become irritable and fly into violent passions. It is always an aggravation of their present complaint. These bursts of temper always aggravate their complaint.

Associated with the lax conditions of the abdominal wall is their liability to sphincter weakness, particularly of the bladder. Most Causticum patients with a cough complain of some urinary incontinence. They are always worse in fresh, clear, bright weather. They are sensitive to cold, sensitive to draught, and better in a soft, moist atmosphere.

Phosphorus

Phosphorus patients typically have a physical appearance similar to Causticum, with delicate features, rather thin faces, fine skin, and slender hands and feet. They may be pale, but the pallor is a different colour from that in Causticum. It is a strange, waxy, transparent pallor. To contrast it – one is the porcelain with the broken glaze, the other is the porcelain with the glaze still on it, which is transparent. That is the type in a Phosphorus who has been ill for years and comes for consultation when acutely ill – either a haemorrhagic patient or one with tuberculosis. But the average Phosphorus patient is absolutely full of vitality. They are alert, very much alive, quick in their movements, bright and intelligent and definitely sensitive; sensitive to their surroundings, to people, to noise, to the atmosphere of the room.

They are tense and restless, quick, impatient and liable to fidget if they are kept waiting. They move their hands or walk about the room – showing the Phosphorus irritability. They have the same explosive anger of Causticum patients, although it is less violent and the after-effects are very different. In Causticum there is an aggravation of their illness; Phosphorus are exhausted and rather ashamed of themselves. Causticum always justify themselves, e.g. people had annoyed them and they were quite right to be angry. Phosphorus are anxious, but it is not the same kind of anxiety as in Causticum, who anticipate trouble particularly for themselves or their relatives. In Phosphorus the anxiety is more a feeling of general dread. They are anxious, nervous and worried, often without being able to say why they are worried. They are tense, and the tension increases in the late afternoon – the twilight aggravation that is mentioned in the Materia Medica. It tends to continue right through the night. Phosphorus patients are afraid of the dark, and all their anxieties tend to persist through the hours of darkness. Almost all Phosphorus are very susceptible to what is called atmosphere, to a sudden drop of the barometer, a thunderstorm or any condition that alters the atmospheric pressure; it may affect their aches and pains, but it always affects them personally.

One helpful point in recognising Phosphorus is that they always have a very variable circulation. During conversation with a Phosphorus patient who is pale, if a sudden idea occurs to him, he colours up at once. Any strong idea makes him colour and he often says that under any excitement he feels his face becoming hot. Any hot or stimulating meal, hot tea or highly seasoned food produces the same effect.

Another point is that, in spite of the fact that they have all this nervous energy and vitality, Phosphorus do become very exhausted. When they are tired they want to keep quiet, their restlessness disappears, they prefer to lie down, and then they like company. Causticum do not mind whether they have anyone near them or not; Phosphorus do. They like sympathy, they are very affectionate, and they are particularly sensitive to certain people. Sometimes Phosphorus have either waking or dreaming premonitions of what is going to happen, which are very often accurate. They say that they have strange feelings on meeting new people – that they have known them before, they know what they are going to say. This type of sensitiveness seems unique to Phosphorus. Another point is that they have almost as much stiffness as Causticum; Causticum patients may develop an acute fibrositis in neck muscles after being out in the cold. Phosphorus have almost the same, but they have a very different reaction. Causticum are not relieved by movement, but Phosphorus can gradually ease the stiffness by movement – massage will help them. Phosphorus patients enjoy being massaged.

Phosphorus have a strong desire for salt. A patient who otherwise appears to need Phosphorus but has no desire for salt should not be given Phosphorus; he might need some Phosphorus compound, but not Phosphorus itself. Phosphorus are worse in damp weather, and much better in a fresh dry atmosphere, as a distinction from Causticum. Phosphorus are aggravated by working in a hot steamy atmosphere.

Phosphorus may be fair or dark and have very lovely hair. There is always a surprising amount of colour and life in their hair, which is fine, whatever the colour. They are never coarse skinned or coarse haired.

Nitric Acid

In appearance, typical Nitric Acid patients are always sallow. They have quite a good colour in their red cheeks, but they look sallow round the eyes. They have dark hair, well-marked eyebrows and soft lips. They are very alive and definite, but have a gloomy outlook. They get intense irritation of the skin, and wounds are slow to heal. They always take a very bad view of the future, and often a very bad view of their attendants too.

They are very obstinate. They are difficult to reason with if they have an idea of their own. Another interesting point is that they have strange appetites. All Nitric Acid patients want pungent-tasting food to stimulate their appetite. They are easily annoyed and get very angry, and will rarely accept an apology. They tend to think people are being unfair to them. They get great amelioration of almost all their symptoms and also of their temper from riding in a car. There is only one exception – a certain number of them tend to get headaches from vibration, which may be brought on in a car that is driven over rough ground. They are always very sensitive to cold.

They are hypersensitive in every way – sensitive to noise, to touch and to pain, and they feel things very acutely.

Normally, Nitric Acid have a strong liking for fats and fatty foods, yet in their digestive disturbances they have an aggravation from taking fats, and this is a point to remember. The only other constant feature is that in any illness they develop a strong odour in the urine.

Medorrhinum

It is not easy to distinguish between Medorrhinum and Thuja patients; their personality, their reactions and their symptoms are so similar. A person who does not respond to Thuja, yet has all the indications for it, will probably be helped with Medorrhinum.

The distinguishing modalities for Medorrhinum are amelioration from lying on the abdomen, amelioration from sea air and a 5 a.m. aggravation.

Lachesis

(The following description is of a person who Dr Borland felt was 'the very essence of Lachesis', Ed.) The patient was a middle-aged woman with reddish-brown hair. She had a very high colour, and the particular point about her colour was the venous engorgement, little veins standing out on her cheeks, little veins standing out on her nose, and a definite bluish appearance of her nose and ears. Her eyes were bright and clear and she was very much alert. Her hands were also rather congested, red, a little swollen and tremulous. She was very restless. In conversation she demonstrated the typical manner in which the Lachesis patient talks – it is very difficult to keep them to the point. It is not that they withhold information, but they do not pay attention to the question. Often they have not got the drift of it, and something else appeals to them and they start off on what they want to say, not on what has been asked. They are at no loss for words, which always stream out of them. She was perfectly frank in telling her tale, and her symptoms were quite well given. On asking about her life and conditions, the outstanding thing was the definite jealousy she had of those members of the family who were well. Her husband was a strong, healthy man who went to business every day and played golf at the weekend, and she was definitely jealous that he was fit and she had to stay in bed. Her daughter was married and had four healthy children. This lady was jealous that her grandchildren were healthy, whereas her own daughters had always been seedy and a worry to her when they were children.

Another typical symptom is that Lachesis are always mixing up the time of day; they think it is evening when it is morning, and morning when it is evening. Another fairly definite characteristic is a very obvious self-consciousness and a weird conceit. In this patient it was mixed up with another typical Lachesis symptom, a very narrow religious outlook. She belonged to some small sect, but she was perfectly certain it was the only sect on the earth; her whole day was spent talking about her religion to those around her, and trying to make them join her own sect. At times she would speak of the amount of money she gave away to keep it going, and it was interesting to note the self-gratification she was getting about it all. At other times she would say that she was a very poor member of the sect and no use to them, and in the next breath, if only she had good health like her husband, she would be able to do so much more. One thing she mentioned was that she had a rather unpleasant experience with her protégés, who had rather done her down. Her husband said that for the past two years his wife had been very suspicious and would give nothing to anyone, even to people she had known for years. He said life was very difficult. He said, 'I don't want to offend my wife because she is not well at present, and one of the things she dislikes is that I should take any alcohol. I am not narrowly religious, but she wants me to keep to her standards. I go out to golf and I want a drink occasionally, and almost the first question I get asked when I come in is, "Have you had a drink?" And she is always wanting to know where I have been and whether I have done anything contrary to her own religious beliefs.'

Another patient has the typical Lachesis suspicion to an even greater degree. She lives in a small village in the country, and is always in trouble because of her suspicion of her neighbours. She is constantly looking for offence and slights, and thinks that people are doing her down – a typical Lachesis reaction.

That is only one type of Lachesis patient. There is another, the chronic alcoholic. They have a more congested appearance than the one that is typical. There is the same tendency to the venous stasis, dilated veins on the face and nose, but not the brightness or the same mental sharpness – the edge of things is a little blunted. There is the same tendency to wander, to half finish one subject and move to the next one. They have the tremor that is frequently present in Lachesis. They are more irritable and much more malicious in their statements about other people than most Lachesis. Lachesis patients are sometimes pale, but the skin is not clear, there are always freckles or congested veins on the face and hands.

Another point about Lachesis alcoholics is that they get a very marked aggravation from food. After food they are more drowsy, more heavy, more muddled, and very liable to get a congested face. They are difficult to treat. Another common reaction in alcoholics is that they are very conscious that they themselves have been responsible for the state they are in, and are very melancholic about it. They are hopeless about anything being done for them, and are very suspicious about any medicine they are given. They think that either it will poison them, or that they are being drugged.

All Lachesis patients have the typical sleep aggravation, i.e. symptoms increase during sleep, so that the patient is worse on waking. They are all very sensitive to heat, and with such congested characteristics they are intolerant of any tightness round them, tight collars, tight belts or anything similar. With any cardiac embarrassment they get very short of breath, want to push the bedclothes down and open the windows.

Ferrum Metallicum
The outstanding feature of Ferrum patients is a very clear skin and, as a rule, a very unstable circulation. They are liable to become pale or to flush on any emotional excitement, exertion, or stimulus of any kind. With the fair skin they have a good colour, particularly over the cheek bones, but very pale mucous membranes. They are definitely anaemic.

They are very easily tired and, without exception, say that if they attempt to hurry they get out of breath, feel absolutely exhausted, and are often faint and giddy. The faintness and giddiness occur with all their complaints, as well as with any over-exertion, talking too much, having to entertain people, or anything similar.

Ferrum patients are very chilly. They feel the cold intensely, usually have very cold extremities, and tend to get very troublesome cramp in their feet. This tends to come on either when they are sitting still or after over-exertion. Another symptom is that they are perfectly all right while going about in the house, but immediately they go out of doors and have to go a little faster, or a little further, they become exhausted.

Mentally, the typical Ferrum condition is a state of depression, despondency and weepiness. In the depression they tend to become confused and anxious, but are unable to give a clear explanation of what is worrying them. Usually they are irritable, particularly from noise, and especially from loud noise.

They are extremely sensitive to pain, may faint if given an injection – yet cannot tolerate any dental work without a local anaesthetic. It is true hyperaesthesia. They appear to be very gentle, pleasant people, a little under the weather, a little depressed, with a pessimistic outlook on life. Yet they simply will not tolerate any opposition, and get into a rage immediately if it is offered. That is one of the main characteristics of Ferrum. They feel exhausted, hot-headed and faint amongst a number of people, and dislike talking to more than one person at a time.

Ferrum and Pulsatilla are rather similar in appearance and temperament, but there is never the intense opposition from Pulsatilla that comes from Ferrum, and their temperature reactions are different. Another symptom often present in Ferrum is constipation. They are always worried by it, and their depression is much more marked when they are constipated.

Ferrum will often clear enuresis in children and may also clear incontinence in the adult.

One other point in connection with Ferrum, a symptom sometimes but not always present, is that they cannot tolerate any dry wine at all, and yet are perfectly all right on a sweet wine. The dry wine gives them a stomach upset and diarrhoea. Chronic diarrhoea that comes on while the patient is actually eating, not after the meal, is a symptom of Ferrum and no other drug. The urging occurs immediately they put anything into their mouths. Ferrum will clear up summer diarrhoea of babies which occurs immediately they begin to feed. A number of remedies have diarrhoea immediately after eating – that is quite common – but only in Ferrum does the diarrhoea occur while eating.

Lycopodium

The typical appearance of Lycopodium patients is that of rather spare, sallow, somewhat wrinkled people. They tend to be dark-haired and, as a rule, are rather above the average height. Usually there is a slight tendency to stoop, and they give the impression of having a long, narrow chest. Sometimes the stoop is more marked in a decidedly thin patient with an almost scaphoid abdomen. They tend to have a worried expression and are a little difficult to get symptoms from. They are rather reticent, and the reticence may become distrust and suspicion, or the reticence may arise from a feeling of diffidence and insecurity. It can happen both ways in Lycopodium. I have never yet met a Lycopodium who was at all expansive. With their very intimate friends they may relax and express their feelings, but they always do it with a certain amount of reservation; they always keep something back and do not give themselves away entirely. As patients this reticence is even more marked, and often gives the impression that they are haughty.

Practically all Lycopodium patients have digestive difficulties. As a rule, they have either jaundiced or muddy conjunctivae, and are lean and livery. They are irritable, peevish and fretful. They want to sit about and be quiet, and dislike being disturbed. They get anxious and apprehensive and dislike being entirely alone, but resent interference. They do not have much stamina and are easily exhausted from either mental or physical exertion. Practically all of them, particularly businessmen, complain that they are exhausted by the end of the afternoon. Their digestion is impaired; they complain of painful flatulence and abdominal distension. After getting home in the evening, if they have an hour's rest and a small meal – they cannot take a big meal because it makes them uncomfortable – they feel much better. That late afternoon aggravation is very constant and agrees with the 4 to 8 p.m. aggravation in all Lycopodium complaints. They are always very slow in the morning. They feel ill and depressed, as if the day's work is going to be too much for them. This occurs at the time they are getting up. After they have had breakfast they feel better, and are confident that they can tackle the day ahead of them.

Associated with the feeling of inability to tackle things is the feeling that their business will not succeed; and, arising out of that, they may become very careful in regard to money matters. They are afraid that they will not have enough to live on, and may become real misers. They are never out-going, are careful with their money, narrow in their outlook, and may become rather intolerant. They have unusual beliefs and ideas, and will not listen to any argument on the subject.

One peculiarity about them is sometimes a little misleading. Although they get a good deal of digestive upset, and practically always get flatulence, and with their flatulence are unable to take a large meal, practically all of them say they cannot manage without food. If they are late for a meal it upsets them. A businessman will say that if he is late for his lunch it upsets him, and yet when he has a meal it has to be a small one.

Lycopodium are very much aggravated by taking any cold food. They have an aggravation from tightness of any kind, particularly around the abdomen, but also a tight hat on the head gives them a headache. They are better from having the head uncovered and from getting out into the fresh air.

One other characteristic point is that they are definitely sensitive to noise, and have a marked hyperaesthesia to any smells, particularly unpleasant smells. A further point is that typical Lycopodium patients do not perspire easily. After strenuous exertion, they may perspire a little and feel better. They tend to have a dry skin, particularly the palms of the hands, which become very hot, burning and uncomfortable. It also occurs on the soles of their feet, particularly from walking about.

Another distinctive feature is that they tend to get a very yellow discolouration of the teeth. It is not due to neglect of the teeth, because many of them are very particular about it. The textbooks say that Lycopodium have a hunger for sweet things, but this is not always present.

Arsenicum Album

One point of contact between Arsenic and Lycopodium is that the typical Arsenicum Alb. patient may occasionally have a miserly tendency. This is the only point of contact between the two remedies – otherwise they are in no way similar. In Arsenicum Alb. the miserliness arises from an entirely different cause. Occasionally it is from a fear of failure, or fear of losing their money, and the over-careful Arsenicum Alb. becomes miserly. The typical cause, however, is covetousness. They appreciate anything beautiful and want to have it. It is more the desire of possession than the fear of poverty. As far as appearance is concerned, typical chronic Arsenicum Alb. people are always very quick, restless, active, intelligent, and alive. They are usually rather finely made. In complexion they tend to be pale, often with dark rings round their eyes, and are usually spare. They have far too much nervous energy, and are too active ever to become really fat.

They are definitely nervous and fussy. They fuss about themselves, they fuss about their health, imagine they have all kinds of diseases, go from one doctor to another, and take up new crazes. They fuss about the family, and are never happy unless they are constantly seeing a doctor. If there is definite opposition to their fussiness, if the members of the family will not go to the doctor, or will not take the latest medicine, then the Arsenicum Alb. patient is very angry with them and is quite sure they will be seriously ill.

They are also fastidious about themselves. They keep themselves neat and tidy, and they like their rooms, bedrooms and their houses very orderly, and are often unduly fussy about it.

Arsenicum Alb. are over-sensitive in every way, to smell, to touch, to light. They are acutely sensitive to cold, and they are liable to get scared and apprehensive if the room gets dark. If there is a noise in the neighbourhood they are afraid it may be burglars. They are always anticipating trouble. They are hypersensitive to tobacco, which makes them very unwell. Many of them suffer from troublesome constipation, and as they are upset almost without exception by fruit and vegetables, it is very difficult to deal with this condition.

I have seen two distinctive types of skin in Arsenicum Alb. patients. In one they have a very fine, smooth skin and very fine hair, and that type usually tends to perspire fairly easily. But there is another Arsenicum Alb. who has a very rough skin, which gets scaly, coarse and unhealthy, and tends to crack. Such people tend to have great difficulty in perspiring; with exertion they get hot and flushed in the face and often develop an acute congestive headache.

Arsenicum Alb. patients sleep badly. They are light sleepers and any noise wakens them about 1 and 2 a.m., and they have a bad nervous spell about that time. Occasionally they will say they never get off to sleep again unless they get up and move about, make some tea or eat something, which often helps them to go to sleep again.

Arsenicum Alb. is frequently indicated in children. They are usually nervy, precocious children who have developed too rapidly and been pushed at school, and if not carefully handled are liable to develop nervous tics. They have nightmares and scream out in the night, they have a terror of the dark and hate to be left alone. Practically always they are very fine-skinned children with fair hair and variable complexion, inclined to be pale yet flushing easily on exertion. They are very restless, the kind of children to whom to sit still is absolute torture. Their skin tends to feel hot and burning rather than itching.

They get definite burning pains, and the surprising thing about the burning pain is that it is relieved by heat, which is exceptional. Lycopodium gets similar burning pains relieved by heat, and it and Arsenicum Alb. are the two remedies that have these pains more than any other. There is one apparent contradiction in Arsenicum Alb. to remember. In connection with their symptoms, they get neuralgic pains. There is intense burning pain in the nerve involved, often the trigeminal, which is relieved by hot applications. They also get congestive headaches accompanied by persistent vomiting. The head feels uncomfortably hot and is relieved by cold applications, or a current of cool air, yet the rest of the body is icy cold. They want the bedclothes up to the neck, they want many blankets and hot bottles, but need their head right by an open window. That is quite different from their neuralgias, where they want hot applications.

Silica

In the textbooks it appears difficult to distinguish Silica and Lycopodium from the mental point of view, and yet Silica and Lycopodium are very different. Typical Silica patients are much more commonly fair-haired. They have a clear skin, never a sallow skin; they usually have a good colour in the cheeks. Very often the skin of the cheeks is a little rough. They tend to have dry lips which crack easily, and they get cracks about the corners of the mouth. If they have nasal catarrh they are liable to get cracks at the corner of the nose. Their hair is fine and they almost always have small bones.

As far as their mentality is concerned, haughtiness never characterises the Silica patient. The typical impression given by Silica is of rather gentle, yielding persons; people who seem as if they would give up very easily. But it is an entirely false impression. They are gentle and polite up to a point, but beyond that they are obstinate, irritable, peevish and most persistent. Silica people are difficult to persuade to take on a job but, if they do take it up, they carry it through to the limit of their ability. They are very conscientious in what they do, and would rather somebody else did it.

Silica children are rather amusing. If handled properly they are very easy to manage. But, if mismanaged, they are just about the most obstinate children it is possible to have, and will often scream and kick.

Both Silica and Lycopodium have a poor memory and from the Materia Medica it is difficult to distinguish them, although in fact they are quite different. In Lycopodium, the tendency to forget is a tendency to forget particular things, like names or something similar. In Silica it is more a question of the patients having had too much to do and the brain being tired and refusing to respond. Thus it is not a lack of memory for individual things, but a tired brain which can take in no more, and cannot remember what it has already learned. Both Lycopodium and Silica are reported as disliking interference. Lycopodium patients want to be left alone, not interfered with or disturbed. In Silica it is much more a matter of disliking personal interference. They do not like to be touched or handled unexpectedly. It makes them jump, and they become annoyed and irritated. If they are depressed and an attempt is made to soothe them, their depression is usually aggravated. They tend to weep, but it does not do them any good. The Lycopodium patient, when depressed, is definitely better from sympathy and understanding. In both remedies the patients are sensitive to cold, but in Lycopodium that sensitiveness to cold is linked up with a definite air hunger, which is not found in Silica.

In both there is an anticipatory dread of undertaking anything. The main distinguishing point about them is that, unless Silica patients are absolutely broken down, although they have a dread of undertaking things, they are capable of doing them well once they start. Lycopodium have a dread of undertaking things and probably make a mess of them.

One thing constant to practically all Silica patients is that under any stress, mental stress or physical exertion they are almost certain to develop a headache, usually a one-sided frontal headache. They may also suffer from recurring headaches which start rather differently. These tend to start in the back of the head, to extend forward and settle in one eye. The stress headache starts over the eye and it may be either eye.

Not only do Silica dislike being touched unexpectedly, even when well, but also they hate jarring of any kind, and commonly get train sick, or develop an acute travel headache, or become generally exhausted by any rough motion.

One other point indicating the possibility of Silica for a patient is that the skin of the finger-tips gets rough, so that it is unpleasant to touch anything. It is a very common Silica symptom; associated with it are cracks round the nails and a tendency to septic fingers. More commonly it is just that roughness of finger-tips which makes it unpleasant to do fine work. It is present even in warm weather, but is more definite if the patient has to have the hands in water frequently.

There is very little to be seen, yet it causes great annoyance. They get deep fissures too, on the tips of the fingers and thumb. If these occur at the sides of the nails they tend to go septic. This is strange, as the typical Silica hand is moist and yet they have this dryness of the finger-tips.

Tuberculinum

It is difficult to get a typical clear-cut picture of Tuberculinum because it may be indicated, at least temporarily, in all sorts of patients. So far as physical make-up is concerned, Tuberculinum is not indicated as a recurring constitutional remedy. Patients may need it occasionally but, as a rule, after it has been given they go on to some other remedy, which they are much more likely to stay on than to revert to Tuberculinum.

However, there is a type of patient that does require a dose of it sometimes. There is one outstanding physical sign which indicates the possibility of Tuberculinum, and this is the peculiar blue colour of the sclera. Apart from that, all sorts of complexions may occur in patients requiring a dose of Tuberculinum.

In children, it has been more commonly indicated in fair children, but in adults all sorts of people may require it. There are certain constant characteristics of Tuberculinum, one of the main indications being a peculiar state of mental restlessness, which is not at all like the Arsenicum Alb. restlessness. It is much more a state of dissatisfaction with their present surroundings and condition, a desire to move about, a desire for change, a desire to go for a holiday, or a desire for travel, anything to alter the present conditions. They are always relieved by motion, whatever their complaint.

Another thing to look for is a change of temperament, from being very good-tempered to being an individual who has become disagreeable, angry or weeping easily. It is a definite change from a previously pleasant disposition. In most Tuberculinum patients, although they have this desire to move about, to see new places and new things, they have a very definite dislike of any mental work. They do physical work quite well, because motion relieves them. This hatred of mental work is linked up with their restlessness; they cannot settle to it.

Another fairly constant symptom in the Tuberculinum state is that they are apt to have acute personal aversions, which have developed recently. A person who has changed, becomes irritable and is developing very definite aversions to individual people, indicates Tuberculinum. Patients with fibrositis which is better from motion, and worse from the cold, require Rhus Tox., whereas if it is better from motion, and worse from heat, they require Tuberculinum. Tuberculinum patients are certainly worse in the heat, but are also aggravated by any sudden change of temperature, whether from cold to hot, or hot to cold, and also any change from dry to damp. Tuberculinum is definitely aggravated in damp cold and in damp hot weather. Rhus Tox is better in warm weather.

Tuberculinum is sometimes very useful in adolescent children. Schoolgirl headaches should respond very well to a dose of Tuberculinum, particularly when dealing with a child who is advanced for her years, bright, intelligent and becoming more irritable than before, becoming nervous of thunderstorms and disliking damp weather, who develops headaches whenever she begins to work, and begins to lose interest in her studies. Tuberculinum is certainly indicated if the child also has a definite fear of dogs.

They are sensitive to music, which often makes them weep, even non-gloomy music. Even though they are so restless, they find standing very exhausting and need to sit down frequently.

Sarsaparilla

There are two, possibly three, types of case with definite indications for Sarsaparilla. The commonest is the one with a definite infection of the urinary tract, in which there is an offensive turbid urine. Clinically the indications for it are either in an infected kidney or cystitis, and there is always a tendency to the formation of calculi, either in the kidney or in the bladder. Associated with the calculus formation are the typical Sarsaparilla modalities. The patient has a certain amount of pain and discomfort on micturition. The pain becomes particularly acute at the end of micturition when the bladder wall contracts either on itself – an inflamed wall – or on a quantity of gritty material in the bladder. The patient feels as if the trouble was actually at the urinary meatus, although it is the bladder contracting down on the calculus that causes the pain. The patient has difficulty in passing urine, which is increased if he or she is lying down. The urine is offensive and there is often a dirty, greyish-greenish deposit.

That is the acute picture. Indications for Sarsaparilla occur occasionally in children with nocturnal enuresis, provided there is a high-smelling urine with a deposit of phosphates and if they tend to get pain on micturition during the day. They have irritating moist eruptions about the genitals where the urine comes in contact with the skin.

Sarsaparilla may also be indicated in skin eruptions. The patients have a marked tendency to skin eruptions of all kinds, but particularly moist excoriating eruptions about the buttocks or the genitals. These are intensely irritating, become raw on scratching and are very much aggravated by washing. Sarsaparilla is the indicated remedy if in addition to the local conditions there is a history of any urinary irritation, particularly if the irritation is most marked at the end of urination, in patients who are sensitive to cold (which distinguishes them from Sulphur) and if the skin irritation is aggravated by any hot stimulating food, such as hot soup.

Sarsaparilla may also be indicated in elderly people with skin eruptions – old patients who look worn and tired and who have an unhealthy wrinkled skin. Very often they have a tendency to varicose veins, their veins stand out on their hands, and they give a history that the skin is difficult to heal after any injury. If they get varicose ulcers they are very slow to heal. They tend to have bluish-coloured stains on the backs of the hands. They are sensitive to cold, particularly cold and damp. They tend to be constipated and are liable to urinary infections. They look rather faded and dirty and they often have a sinking feeling in the abdomen, not associated with hunger, just an uncomfortable empty feeling. They are the kind of people that seem to need Sulphur. Yet mentally and physically they improve on Sarsaparilla.

Occasionally, younger patients with very severe dysmenorrhoea will be helped by Sarsaparilla. They have extreme pain in the back and the lower abdomen, extending down the thighs, which completely incapacitates them and which is associated with faintness, perspiring, vomiting and diarrhoea. With the dysmenorrhoea they tend to have very acute mammary sensitiveness, often one-sided; the left side is more commonly involved than the right. They also get a very distinctive headache. They have a sensation as if they had a tight band right round the head, from the occiput to the forehead. The headache is much worse from any pressure and is often associated with a feeling of fullness and possibly actual swelling of the bridge of the nose. These cases respond very well to Sarsaparilla.

That description will indicate the relationships of Sarsaparilla. Patients who need Sarsaparilla for acute conditions frequently have indications for Sulphur or Sepia. Patients with skin conditions need the Sulphur-Sarsaparilla follow-on. Dysmenorrhoea patients have their acute Sarsaparilla symptoms and very often, once the acute stage is over, there are indications for Sepia, which is the Sarsaparilla-Sepia follow-on.

The Psorinum picture is almost identical with that of Sarsaparilla, particularly in old people.

Sanicula

Sanicula is one of the most valuable remedies in the Materia Medica, and in a very large number of cases Silica is prescribed where Sanicula should be given. There are certain clear distinguishing points between Silica and Sanicula, and Sanicula seems to be rather wider in its action than Silica. Sanicula is more often needed for patients with skin eruptions than Silica.

The picture of Sanicula in children and in adults is rather different. In children the typical Sanicula make-up is one of intense irritability. They are very restless and active. They are intensely irritable, extremely obstinate, and they hate being handled. Patients requiring Sanicula are very similar in character to those who benefit from Chamomilla. Sanicula children have a very marked aggravation from downward motion. Chamomilla children enjoy being rocked and tossed about. Sanicula children shriek immediately they are moved downward. Chamomilla children hate to be left alone because they want attention; Sanicula children hate to be touched and resist it, and are also terrified in the dark. As a rule, Sanicula children want to be fed all the time, and yet they cannot digest what they eat. After being fed, they vomit almost immediately, no matter what food they have been given – milk, water, barley water – and immediately want to be fed again. They have a marked time of aggravation from about 9 p.m. until some time after midnight. Sanicula children are almost always constipated. They sometimes have an attack of diarrhoea, with the variation in the colour and consistency of the stool that is characteristic of Sanicula. Whether they are constipated or whether suffering from diarrhoea, there is always intense straining to stool.

With acute digestive upsets, Sanicula children tend to have a very dry mouth with painful, hot, ulcerated patches on the tongue, particularly on the under surface. This tendency to ulceration of the mouth may also occur in adults, and these ulcerated patches are acutely sensitive.

Sanicula children tend to perspire freely. The typical textbook description is that the children perspire about the back of their head, but actually they perspire on the part of the body they are lying on. If they are lying on their back, the back of their head perspires, but they also perspire all down the back. In adults, if they are lying in bed with their hands on the chest, the under surface of the arm where it is in

contact with the chest is damp, or the side of the head and be
lain on.

Sanicula patients tend to have unhealthy skins. The hands ,
perspire, the perspiration is often offensive, and yet in spite ., the
moisture they tend to have cracks on the backs of the hands, which
bleed and are sensitive. They get eczema on the fingers, and tend to
develop eczematous eruptions round the backs of the ears. All these
eruptions have a similar discharge to that found in Graphites or
Petroleum – a sticky, yellowish discharge which is offensive.

The perspiration of Sanicula is both offensive and excoriating. It
makes their feet raw and rots their socks and sometimes even their
shoes.

Although the extremities feel cold and clammy to touch, these
children constantly put their feet out of bed at night. Their feet get very
hot and burning, perspire and are extremely offensive.

As far as likes and dislikes are concerned, one thing that helps to
distinguish between Sanicula and Silica children is that Sanicula
children like ice-cold milk, and Silica children mostly dislike milk in
any form. Sanicula also have a definite craving for salty things, bacon
particularly, or actual salt.

These children often have sticky eye discharges and they have a very
marked photophobia, often without any obvious eye lesion at all or with
very little inflammatory disturbance in the eye. Linking up with the
sticky eye discharge, they very often have a troublesome nasal
discharge, a crusty nasal discharge, with a scabby, scaly eruption on
the upper lip. They are very frightened of the dark.

Usually these children are under-nourished, underweight, very thin
about the neck, and often have a distended abdomen. They tend to have
enuresis. In other words, the 'pot-bellied' marasmic child is often a
Sanicula child and not a Silica.

Adult Sanicula patients are more interesting. They are very like
Silica. Their main complaint is of a feeling of complete exhaustion.
They say that they feel so exhausted that the mere thought of work is
impossible, they feel all they want to do is to lie down and go to sleep.
With that feeling of exhaustion they are usually depressed, they have a
sense of dread, a feeling of impending trouble, although it is not usually
very definite. Another characteristic is that they have a marvellous
faculty for misinterpreting what is being done for them.

They practically always suffer from headaches, and the Sanicula
headaches are very typical. The pain usually starts in the back of the
neck just below the occiput, and spreads right up over the head and

settles in the forehead. The patients are acutely sensitive to any cold or draught; going out into the cold air will very often bring on the headache or, if already present, will make it very much worse. During the headache the pain is aggravated by any exertion, any motion, light or noise, and is usually associated with a certain amount of photophobia. Associated with the tiredness, one of the marked Sanicula characteristics is a pain in the lumbosacral region. It is a completely crippling pain and it has definite modalities. Patients are usually fairly free of pain in the morning after a night's rest, and it gradually develops during the day. While it is bad they feel completely exhausted and want to lie down. The pain is relieved by pressure and lying on the back. As the day advances, the pain tends to ease up and has usually disappeared by evening round about 6, 7 or 8 p.m.

Sanicula also have an arthritic condition of the shoulder joints, particularly marked on the right side. It is worthwhile linking this with the back condition, because while their back is bad any attempt to use their arms increases the pain; and while the shoulder region is involved it is completely impossible for the patient to put the arm behind his back. They are unable to put on their coat, and find it almost impossible to raise the arm up to the head. The pain is usually situated just in the top of the shoulder. Patients with shoulder pain who need Ferrum have practically the same modalities, except that they are eased by moving the arm gently, although they have the same limitation of movement. In Ferrum the pain is relieved by gentle motion; Sanicula are not relieved by motion at all.

These tired out patients have a very slow digestion. After a meal they do not want any more food for six or eight hours. If they eat anything sooner, they may vomit. Associated with their slow digestion is the most obstinate constipation. They are uncomfortable with it and feel that their bowels want to act, and there is intense straining. The stools are very small in size and usually hard. Alumina and Silica patients have a similar type of constipation – a great effort and very little result. The stool is usually in hard lumps.

Another useful point about Sanicula is that they tend to have a dry scaly eruption on the eyebrows. A similar condition is seen in Phosphorus. Remember that Sanicula are sensitive to cold and have a desire for salt. They have this general weariness and this scaly eruption on the eyebrows. All these symptoms are also found in Phosphorus, so that it is important to distinguish between them.

There are two other points. One is that Sanicula are very sensitive to motion. They get violent headaches and become sick from any journey, and they are particularly sensitive to the motion of going down in a lift.

The other point is that they tend to sleep very badly, with most distressing dreams. The dreams are of two types. One is a dream of burglars in the house. It is so vivid and real that they sometimes must get out of bed and go round the house to make sure that there is no one there before they can settle down and go to sleep again. The other is a dream of murder; either they themselves are being murdered, or they are committing murder.

One other mental characteristic Sanicula patients have, which is the same as in children, is a marked dislike of the dark, particularly of going out and walking in the dark. They are thoroughly scared, and have a feeling that there is someone behind them. They do not get this feeling during the day; only in the dark. Sepia have the same feeling, but in the daytime as well. Medorrhinum have it during the dark too, and also the dreams of robbers. But Sanicula only have it when out in the dark.

Chapter 13

Comparison of Lilium Tigrinum, Natrum Muriaticum and Sepia

In comparing Lilium Tig., Natrum Mur. and Sepia patients one notes various impressions as they come into the consulting room. It is a little difficult to place Lilium Tig. in appearance. The first thing to realise is that they are fairly compact and full-blooded, and the majority of them fair rather than dark. They are determined personalities, not soft and yielding, yet not taut like Natrum Mur., and different from the resentful attitude often present in Sepia. They tend to be fat rather than thin, and definitely hot-blooded. If they enter a hot room they loosen their coat immediately and prefer to keep away from any source of heat. They tend to be slightly cyanotic. Their lips are often quite dark in colour and usually pretty full.

The Natrum Mur. patient always strikes one as being a very definite character. The description in textbooks as being a thin patient is not true in many cases. Children are thin but adults are well-covered; women especially tend to be broad, but they are usually thin-necked, surprisingly so for their build. Their hair may be any colour from sandy to dark brown, not usually black. Their skin is always sallow, but very often when they come into the consulting room they are excited and flushed. This rather high colour masks the sallowness and may cause them to be confused with Phosphorus, who have a malar flush. Looking at them they appear quite intelligent, quite alive.

Their movements are fairly short, rapid and definite. It is an effort for them to consult a doctor. Their carotid pulsation will show that their pulse rate is accelerated, and their hands tremble. With this excitement there is a tendency for their skin to become rather oily – it only occurs under excitement or if the room is hot. If the patient has recently had a cold, almost certainly there will be a herpes about the lips. The textbooks state that Natrum Mur. patients are anaemic but quite a number have very red lips, and there is very often a crack in the lower or upper lip, about the centre.

Consider Sepia patients as a contrast. They may be fair or dark-haired, and are more often women than men. They come resentfully. There are two types – either the patient comes because she has been sent and resents it, or she resents being ill and having to talk about it. Usually she gives no pleasant word of greeting and as a rule enters with a sullen expression.

The next impression is the rather stupid expression, which may be caused by stupidity, tiredness or a slow-acting brain. It may be any of them. In contrast with Natrum Mur., the Sepia patient's face is often fatter than expected – quite often the person is thin in body, above average height, yet in spite of their thinness elsewhere, the face is fat. Their colour is a quite distinct sallow not seen in any other remedy. It is especially noticeable round the eyes and is a peculiar brownish pigmentation spreading out on to the nose and cheek bones. Possibly she will have a wart somewhere and almost always it is brownish in colour, especially after 40 years of age. The Sepia patient is generally pale and almost always has pale lips. The next thing to notice is the way they sit down in the chair. They sink into it. They are tired. Natrum Mur. sit on the edge of the chair and get annoyed if asked questions. The one is taut, the other relaxed. There is one point that suggests Natrum Mur. – the first appearance is of a very tidy and neat, trim patient, but on looking closer they are not nearly as tidy as they seem to be. Phosphorus is always scrupulously tidy and so is Arsenicum Alb., but not Natrum Mur.

MENTALITIES

Lilium Tig., Natrum Mur. and Sepia patients are all aggravated by consolation, but there are differences. The Lilium Tig. reaction to consolation is definitely bad-tempered. They have all sorts of strange ideas, that people are annoying them deliberately, and any sympathy or attempted explanation only increases their annoyance. The Natrum Mur. reaction to consolation is quite different, particularly when depressed. When they are ill and depressed and anyone consoles them they break down and weep. They do not display the same irritability as Lilium Tig. The Sepia aggravation from consolation is again quite distinct. They have a general resentment against their fate, think that they have had a poor deal in life and are tired out, and if consolation is given they will turn on the giver. They are physically worn out, depressed and weak, they develop a headache and if consoled start weeping. It is, however, different from Natrum Mur.; Natrum Mur. gets relief from weeping but Sepia is always worse if she has wept.

There are other differences. The main characteristic of Lilium Tig. is their irritability – it is almost impossible to please them. They are most exacting; they want everything to centre round themselves, and if it does not they fly into a rage. There is often a certain amount of fear associated with their complaints, and they are very likely to develop fear of insanity. They also have the idea that they have some undiagnosed disease, which they feel is always undiagnosed through lack of knowledge on the part of the physician who is looking after them, and they have a dread of it. With these bad tempers, after a spell where everyone has tried to please them, they go on to a religious phase of remorse. They become tearful, depressed and generally indifferent to their surroundings. With Lilium Tig. patients, the phrasing of the questions and the wording of the advice given must be carefully chosen, as they will take it as criticism of what they have done previously rather than as advice for the future. If there is a possibility of taking anything the wrong way they will always do so.

Contrast this with Natrum Mur. and there is a great difference. Natrum Mur. are either depressed or excited, never anything for long at a time, a weird mixture. There is an absolute lack of a sense of humour; they are often laughing and often weeping, but a pure sense of fun is simply lacking. They are also very difficult to get on with. They crave attention yet, if it is given, they are just about as disagreeable as they can be. They resent it if they do not get it, and are dissatisfied if they do. Impatience is a very marked characteristic. They want a thing done at once or not at all. They are very much upset by excitement and extraordinarily sensitive to noise, particularly to sudden noises. If anyone is in a room when a Natrum Mur. patient is reading, and fidgets or moves about, it makes them extremely irritable. They have a strange susceptibility to music. All Natrum salts have it, but especially Natrum Mur. They are sensitive to some types of music only, as they are not really musical, but are especially sensitive to sentimental music which they really enjoy, while serious music causes no reaction. They remember every slight they have ever had. If an explanation is given they forget the explanation and remember the original idea. They are excellent haters. They are most difficult people to live with, though often very pleasant to meet.

Almost the same terms are used in the textbooks with regard to Sepia, yet they are as different as night from day. Sepia has about as much excitement and intolerance to noise, yet the whole mentality is different. Sepia is a tired-out patient, nervously, mentally and physically. They do a good deal of weeping, but it is a sort of despairing weeping. They feel defeated and that they cannot go on, and sit down and weep. As a rule, any attempt to encourage them puts them into an obstinate and resentful mood, thinking they are martyrs and that people have not been fair to them. In this exhausted state they tend to become melancholy. They dislike to be spoken to or interfered with; they do not want anyone to help them out or to make them well. That is the characteristic Sepia mentality, but occasionally they may become more excitable if under stress, becoming apprehensive and developing illogical fears. Worries become exaggerated, and they fear that something dreadful is going to happen, or that they are becoming insane. If their husband is ill they dread disaster. They say that they have always been independent and now they are heading for charity. This is more the dread of dependency than of poverty. When they are tired out they become envious of people who are not having such a bad time, and they are very spiteful in their remarks about them.

GENERAL REACTIONS

In the general temperature reactions of these three remedies there is apparent similarity and a real difference. All three have intolerance of warm, stuffy rooms, but there the similarity ceases. Lilium Tig. have definite aggravation in heat, are much worse in a stuffy room and develop headaches and breathlessness from it. They are always better from moving about, particularly from moving about out of doors. The one exception to this amelioration from movement is when they are suffering from actual uterine prolapse. In all three remedies there is a marked tendency to symptoms of prolapse, even without actual uterine displacement. Natrum Mur. have aggravation in a warm room but are aggravated by both heat and cold. They do not stand heat well and are intolerant of the sun. On the other hand, they cannot stand draughts and are sensitive to extreme cold, and often suffer from cold and numb extremities.

Incidentally, Lilium Tig. patients have warm extremities and might be confused with Sulphur patients, especially as they also have the early morning 'Sulphur diarrhoea'. Sepia has a definite aggravation in a warm room, which causes faintness. They are liable to faint if standing or kneeling for too long. They do not stand cold well in any form, yet stuffiness upsets them. They often have cold damp extremities and often have an offensive foot sweat. They are very sensitive to weather, cold damp weather, or a change from cold to warm or from dry to wet. Natrum Mur. and Sepia have a definite aggravation from thunder, but Sepia have a desperate fear, much more marked than Natrum Mur.

Lilium Tig. are better from walking about in the open air. Sepia are better if they exert themselves enough to warm them up. Natrum Mur., on the other hand, are aggravated by exercise which is strenuous enough to make them hot. There is one point which is very often a useful differentiating one – the mid-morning aggravation of Natrum Mur., which the other two remedies do not have. It is round about 10 to 11 a.m., when all their symptoms tend to be worse. Lilium Tig. patients have early morning aggravation; Sepia have a general morning aggravation. If Sepia have a good night's sleep they feel better, but after only a short sleep they almost certainly waken with a severe headache and feel as if they are going to die.

HEADACHE

Headaches are quite different in the three remedies. A typical Lilium Tig. headache is a frontal one with mental confusion. The patients say they feel half crazy. There is ocular disturbance, and if the headache is very severe they may develop an internal strabismus. The headache may extend down the back of the neck. One interesting point is that they often develop abdominal disturbance, especially pain in the right iliac fossa, associated with their headaches. Natrum Mur. headaches are very different. There are two types. In the first, the patient wakes up with slight headache in the morning and it increases all day. It is a very severe headache and is usually associated with the menstrual period, coming just before or just after. In the second type, the headache comes on during mid-morning, 10 to 11 a.m., and eases off about 4 p.m. This is a sun headache increasing and decreasing with the heat of the sun, at its maximum when the sun is strongest and disappearing about sunset. There is a certain amount of ocular disturbance associated with the Natrum Mur. headaches. The patients are exceedingly sensitive to light, their eyes become hot and tired, and smart with pain which increases from any attempt to use the eyes for close work, like reading or sewing.

The Sepia headache on the other hand usually starts in morning. If severe it tends to get worse till early in the evening, when the patient is likely to vomit. There is a feeling of intense congestion all over the head. One distinguishing feature between Natrum Mur. and Sepia headaches is that Sepia tend to be relieved by applied heat; not so Natrum Mur. Both are bad in a stuffy room. Also in Sepia the headache is relieved by hard pressure, and they often tie the head up tight. Both Natrum Mur. and Sepia are aggravated by jarring or any movement.

FOOD

Patients requiring any of these three remedies tend to be hungry. Lilium Tig. probably have the biggest appetites. Occasionally, there is complete loss of appetite in any of the remedies, but usually the patients have big appetites. Lilium Tig. remain hungry in spite of having had a good meal. Natrum Mur. are hungry but have no capacity, and are very soon satiated. Sepia have a feeling of emptiness which is not relieved by food; it is an artificial feeling of hunger. Lilium Tig. dislike coffee and sometimes bread, although by no means constantly, but they do have a very strong dislike for meat. Natrum Mur. have quite marked food idiosyncrasies. They like salt, often in excess, like all Natrums. They like bitter foods, such as beer, and often like fish very much, but have a definite aversion to fat food. Natrum Mur. often have an aggravation from sour wine, and dislike tobacco. Sepia have a definite intolerance for tobacco, it makes them sick; the smell of cooking also makes them feel sick. They have a definite dislike for meat and milk, and a liking for spicy foods. They have also a peculiar desire for vinegar and stimulants, possibly in order to stimulate a jaded appetite.

ABDOMINAL

Lilium Tig. is typical of the fat well-nourished abdominal neurasthenic, like a woman with a sensation as if everything in the abdomen were dragging down. This is so marked that she will very often apply support to the perineum because she feels everything is coming out. She feels as if the whole abdominal contents were dropping down. In spite of her relief from supporting the abdomen she has a peculiar sensitiveness to any pressure in the epigastrium, which makes her feel sick. The most common displacement in Lilium Tig. is an anteversion of the uterus;

associated with this there is a sensation of something pressing into the rectum and an urgent desire for the bowels to act. With the displacement there is a good deal of pelvic congestion and marked sexual excitement. The periods are scanty, commonly the flow stops when in bed and only starts again on getting up in the morning and moving about. Natrum Mur. patients do not have the severe dragging sensation. They have irregular periods which may last a day or may last a week, may be excessive or may be scanty, but are extremely variable. All complaints are aggravated at the period time, it may be during or after, but occasionally may be before. The most common form of disturbance is backache, especially in the morning, and getting better when the patient is up and moving about. They tend to develop general backache. This is generally aggravated by moving about and better from pressure, especially from lying down on something hard. Sepia patients have almost as much drag as Lilium Tig., but not so widely spread. They feel all their pelvic contents coming down, but not the whole abdominal contents. The typical Sepia patient is the kind of woman who has had half a dozen children, all close together, possibly with some pelvic infection. They may have any displacement, but the common one is a retroversion, though they may have a prolapse. Lilium Tig. patients feel as if there is a lump in the rectum, with tenesmus. In Sepia patients there is not much tenesmus, but they feel the bowel is full and they have a moist oozing from the anus. During the menstrual period they have a very acute sacral pain and they may get a certain amount of backache, but not so marked as in Natrum Mur. The ache is relieved by movement, and immediately they rest it recurs. It is relieved by pressure, but never by lying down on something hard, as in Natrum Mur. This is a differentiating point.

SEXUAL

There is one final point in which the three remedies show strongly marked differences, namely in their sexual relationships.

In Lilium Tig. there is marked sexual over-excitability, sometimes even to a pathological degree. In the other two remedies there is a definite aversion to sexual relationships. In Natrum Mur. this is commonly because sexual intercourse is often extremely painful, owing to the dry state of the vaginal mucous membranes, this dryness of the mucous membranes being a very general symptom in Natrum Mur. In Sepia there is a sexual coldness; they are tired out physically, they often have a dread of further pregnancy, and in many cases there is an aversion to the husband.

Chapter 14

The Use of Four Nosodes

Consider using a nosode in any illness, whether acute or chronic, where there are definite clear indications for a remedy, and where it does not produce the effect that is justifiably expected. Dealing with an acute case, in the normal way, if the improvement lasts a few hours the chosen remedy is repeated and is again effective. It is purely a question of spacing the doses. There are a certain number of cases in which repeated doses of the apparently indicated remedy do not give the expected effect – these are the ones which call for a nosode.

If the condition is sub-acute, and the clearly indicated remedy helps the patient for only ten days or so rather than the expected four to five weeks, that is nevertheless within the normal range of reaction. The remedy should be repeated either in the same or a higher potency. If instead of improving the symptoms for ten days it holds for a fortnight or a little longer, that is a perfectly satisfactory response. But if, on repeating in a higher potency, the effect of the remedy again only lasts a week or ten days and the patient's symptoms are returning, or becoming worse, a nosode is indicated. Similarly in a chronic case, if the effect of the remedy lasts two or three weeks, with the same sort of response to the repeated or higher potency, a nosode is required.

There are one or two other conditions which interfere with the action of the remedies and which shorten the effective length of action of the dose. In both acute and chronic cases the commonest cause is a hidden septic focus of some kind. In acute cases after an operation, where there may be the beginning of a stitch abscess or a deep-seated infected blood clot, the infection may interfere with the action of the remedy. This may occur in chest conditions where the patient is developing a small empyema, occasionally in ear infections where there is mastoid involvement or in a dental abscess.

It is necessary to eliminate the presence of a septic focus before prescribing a nosode, because a septic focus in either an acute or chronic case does interfere with the action of the remedy. In a chronic case there is also a possibility that the patient has been put on a remedy which is antidoted by one of the common foods. Quite a number of drugs are antidoted by coffee. These food aggravations are listed in the Repertory – if the indicated remedy is not in that list it can be ignored. If it is present in first or second type, the patient should be warned against taking the particular article of diet as long as he is on that remedy. (*Note.* First type in the Repertory is heavy black type and indicates a well proved reaction – second type is italic and indicates a less well proved reaction. Ed.)

The most difficult decision to make is which of the nosodes is required, and this depends to a large extent on the actual symptoms given by the patient. Unfortunately, there is a percentage of cases which do not give clear indications for any particular nosode.

If there are indications for one particular nosode, then there is no difficulty. Without clear indications, the choice lies between Psorinum, Tuberculinum, Medorrhinum and Syphilinum. That was entirely true until the bowel nosodes were introduced into homoeopathic practice. The kind of case likely to need a bowel nosode is one where there is a low grade toxaemia, chronic mild headaches, chronic mild digestive upsets, chronic fibrositis and occasionally disturbance of thyroid secretion. If such a case does not respond to treatment, it is advisable to have a series of stool examinations. An isolated stool examination is useless – the seat of maximum growth of these bowel organisms is in the small intestine, not the large intestine. It is necessary to use liquid material from the small intestine, or the culture will be negative. If there is no access to a laboratory, a polyvalent bowel nosode can be used.

In the majority of cases requiring a bowel nosode, indications for Sulphur have usually been present. Kali Carb. is the next most commonly indicated remedy where the expected reaction has not occurred and where a nosode may be needed. A bowel nosode may be required when indications for any Potassium salt have been present. The next most common remedies are the Silver salts, either Argentum Nit. or Argentum Met. After these, the cases in which bowel nosodes may be required are digestive ones giving indications for Lycopodium, Graphites, Anacardium or Chelidonium. In each case the expected improvement has not taken place and a nosode may be required.

Of the four nosodes first mentioned – Psorinum, Tuberculinum, Medorrhinum and Syphilinum – the commonest is Psorinum.

Psorinum

The main indication for Psorinum is the state of general sluggishness of the whole body. The patients have a very poor resistance to acute disease, and there has been a progressive decrease of vitality in the chronic case. They are always tired, have no energy, have a poor circulation, and are sensitive to cold. They have a poor skin reaction that is shown either in the form of a very unhealthy looking skin with a greasy surface, or a tendency to pimples, boils and skin eruptions of all kinds. Practically all Psorinum patients have what they describe either as hunger or emptiness. With some of them it is actual hunger, and with others it is just a feeling of emptiness and sinking in the abdomen. This describes the case where there are no characteristic Psorinum indications. These are the indefinite indications which are present in a patient who is giving no clear prescribing symptoms at all, and that is the kind of case for Psorinum. Naturally, the remedy which has already been prescribed in such cases is one indicated for patients with a lowered vitality, and the commonest is probably Sepia. Think of all the chilly drugs in which the patient has a lowered vitality – Sepia, Silica, Phosphorus, Phosphoric Acid, Lycopodium, Calcarea. Those are the types in which an intercurrent dose of Psorinum may be required.

Tuberculinum Bovinum

Probably the next most common nosode to be required is Tuberculinum. It is imperative to remember that the Tuberculinum temperature reaction is very definite. Tuberculinum patients are sensitive to extreme heat and particularly sensitive to any lack of oxygen in the atmosphere. They may be chilly in themselves.

Constant in all Tuberculinum patients is the fact that they are better from moving about. They may be very tired, but if they move about gently it does help them. They may get more tired after exertion, and any violent exertion that heats them up will certainly exhaust them, but gently moving about – no matter what their complaint – does ease them.

They also tend to lose weight, are mostly thin or at least underweight, and are over-sensitive to atmospheric changes.

Considering these indications, it is quite easy to see the type of remedy in which an intercurrent dose of Tuberculinum might be required. Any of the hot-blooded drugs might require it. For instance an acute Apis case very often needs a dose of Tuberculinum during convalescence; Argentum Nit. also quite frequently need intercurrent doses of Tuberculinum; the Baryta Mur. patient with repeated sore throats is another case. Often these throat infections can be stopped altogether with an intercurrent dose of Tuberculinum – it does not have the same effect on the Baryta Carb. who is a chilly patient.

A certain number of patients who are Arsenicum Alb. but who do not have the Arsenicum Alb. chilliness, if given Arsenicum Iodide do very well indeed, up to a point; these Arsenicum Iodide patients mostly need a dose of Tuberculinum sooner or later. A Calcarea Carb. child, who has responded to the remedy and becomes less sensitive to cold, is very often improved by an intercurrent dose of Tuberculinum when he is not making any further progress. It is much more common in the Calc. Phos. child, who is thinner, and commoner still in the Calc. Sulph. child or adult, that an intercurrent dose of Tuberculinum is required. Not infrequently it is indicated in Lycopodium types and also in those requiring the Natrum salts, with the possible exception of Natrum Carb. Very frequently, indications for an intercurrent dose of Tuberculinum may occur in Sulphur and in Pulsatilla types.

There is one exception to the normal Tuberculinum temperature reaction. With a history of tuberculosis in the family – not in the individual patient – and where the patient is chilly, despite the chilliness they respond very well to an intercurrent dose of Tuberculinum, particularly in the Phosphorus or Silica type of patient.

In cases where Tuberculinum is used as an intercurrent remedy, after a single dose, prescribe the original remedy after an interval and the patient should progress for months. Tuberculinum has to be repeated more frequently than other remedies when prescribed as an indicated remedy on its particular indications. It has to be repeated in about three weeks. A certain number of patients with symptoms similar to those of Rhus Tox., but with temperature reactions altered, need Tuberculinum. However, the effect rarely lasts more than three weeks without a repetition.

Medorrhinum
There are two types of case in which to look for Medorrhinum indications. The first and commonest is the patient with a chronic catarrhal chest, whether with or without asthmatic attacks. The next commonest is the patient with fibrositis. In the majority of catarrhal chest conditions with Medorrhinum indications, the patients complain of chronic laryngeal irritation, either a laryngeal cough or a tendency to hoarseness or sensitiveness of the voice. In patients with indications for remedies like Natrum Sulph., Argentum Nit., Kali Sulph., Causticum or Sepia, in a chest condition – chronic bronchitis or bronchitis with

asthma – a dose of Medorrhinum is almost always required sometime during the course of treatment. When dealing with a fibrositic or an arthritic condition in patients with indications for Apis, Calcarea, Ferrum, Fluoric Acid, Manganese, Phytolacca or Thuja, again look for Medorrhinum indications.

Syphilinum (Lueticum)

The last of the common nosodes is Syphilinum. There are certain types of cases with indications for Syphilinum, apart from a definite syphilitic history. But where there is a syphilitic history, particularly in the parents of the patient, it is more than probable that a dose of Syphilinum will be needed in the course of treatment. Where there is a syphilitic history in the patient himself, with the story that the syphilis has been effectively treated and he now has a negative Wassermann, Syphilinum is also very likely to be required.

In some patients there may be indications for Syphilinum apart from an actual history of syphilis. The commonest is a catarrhal condition of the upper respiratory passages, chronic nasal catarrh, particularly where the catarrh tends to produce an atrophic condition of the mucous membrane, with a certain amount of bleeding – the patient who says he gets a crusty condition of the nose. It is a case which is very obstinate to treat, but there is a response to a dose of Syphilinum quite apart from a syphilitic history. Occasionally a dose of Syphilinum sets up a reaction and improvement in a granular pharyngitis which is not responding to treatment.

The next most common case is recurring iritis, not necessarily syphilitic, which often responds well to Syphilinum.

Indications for Syphilinum may occur in arthritic cases, such as rheumatoid arthritis. In these rheumatic cases there is a guide to prescribing from the remedy which the patient has been on previously. Syphilinum often helps in an arthritic patient who has been requiring Arsenicum Alb. and any of the Aurum salts, Aurum Met., Aurum Chlor. or Aurum Sulphide; any of these patients may give indications for Syphilinum. All the Kali salts – Kali Bich., Kali Ars. and, more than any other possibly, Kali Sulph. – in rheumatic conditions often give indications for Syphilinum. There may also be indications for Syphilinum where any of the Mercurius preparations have been used. It may be needed in a case that has had benefit from Nitric Acid. Rheumatic cases that have responded to Phytolacca very often progress to Mercurius and then on to Syphilinum. Sometimes it may benefit typical Silica patients – Silica arthritics – who have had some improvement which has not persisted, and after an intercurrent dose of Syphilinum they will continue to make progress.

Some ulcers of the legs that have the typical appearance of Carbo Veg., the sluggish, atrophic ulcers, respond to Syphilinum although there is no syphilitic history. A certain number of these ulcers also respond to Tuberculinum or Psorinum.

The improvement following a nosode usually lasts for 2–3 weeks. If there are definite indications for one particular nosode, it may be given in a high potency, otherwise it is best to use a 30c.

The Biochemic System of Medicine
WHAT IT IS, HOW IT WORKS, WHAT IT DOES

Dr. Wilhelm Heinrich Schuessler was one of the outstanding intellects of the last century and a man whose scientific vision was far ahead of his time. He created the Biochemic System of Medicine.

He postulated that inorganic matter — essential to health and, indeed, to life itself — was comprised of twelve principal "tissue salts" and that a deficiency, or imbalance, of any of these would create ill-health.

He stated that when the deficiency was corrected the cells again functioned normally and health was restored.

The fundamental basis of the Biochemic System of Medicine is the twelve tissue salts which he isolated. These are now available in tablet form and are known by NUMBERS and also by distinctive abbreviated names. They have specific actions, one for the blood, another for the skin, and so on.

Research by New Era Laboratories then turned its attention to specific ailments and illnesses. From that research came the production of eighteen "Combination" remedies to be used in the treatment of a variety of everyday ailments. The ailments are clearly stated on the packs, and the individual **New Era**® Combinations are known by LETTERS.

The latest development is the preparation of six further remedies for specified ailments.

The twelve **New Era**® Tissue Salts, the eighteen **New Era**® Combination Remedies and the six latest remedies are all incorporated in the form of small, moulded lactose-based tablets, homoeopathically prepared. The tablets are moulded (not compressed) so that they dissolve in the mouth and hence are absorbed quickly through the membranes of the mouth and tongue and so into the blood stream. They are therefore available to the body quite quickly.

New Era® Biochemic Remedies are extremely safe, gentle, natural remedies. Apart from the very rare case of those who suffer from lactose (milk sugar) intolerance, the normal dosage, or even considerable over-dosage, presents no risk of side effects. What is more, they do not mask symptoms of ailments they cannot treat. They leave them alone so that sufferers *know* they must seek specific medical advice.

Additional to the tabletted remedies, there is also a range of Biochemic Skin Balms using combinations of Tissue Salts in ointment bases.

The **New Era**® Biochemic Remedies are unique in that no other Company in the world possesses Product Licences of Right for products formulated in accordance with the Schuessler System and produced in premises properly licensed and inspected.

This leaflet is intended merely to introduce the Biochemic System of Medicine. Much has been written on the system and your retailer will be able to supply you with explanatory leaflets and recommend suitable books, particularly the inexpensive "A Guide to Biochemic Tissue Salts" by Dr. Andrew Stanway, MB, MRCP. Or write to New Era.

**NEW ERA LABORATORIES LIMITED,
39 WALES FARM ROAD, LONDON W3 6XH**

This product — **NEW ERA**® REMEDY No. 6 — is a Tissue Salt within the Biochemic System of Medicine.

SOME FACTS ABOUT NERVY AND EDGY CONDITIONS

The trials and tribulations of everyday life can sometimes make the calmest person feel nervy and edgy. Worry or excitement can cause feelings of stress and strain.

At such times **New Era**® Tissue Salt No. 6 (Kali. Phos. 6×) is the one to turn to. Like all **New Era**® tissue salts, it is safe and easy to use and since it has no side effects it can be used with confidence by people of all ages.

Remedy Index